Nifast
Communications for Healthcare

Communications for Healthcare

FETAC Level 5

Nifast

Consultant editor: Anita Duffy

Gill & Macmillan

Gill & Macmillan
Hume Avenue, Park West, Dublin 12
www.gillmacmillan.ie

© Nifast 2015

978 07171 5728 0

Consultant editor: Anita Duffy
Design and print origination by Síofra Murphy
Printed by GraphyCems, Spain

For permission to reproduce photographs, the author and publisher gratefully acknowledge the following:

© Library of Congress Prints and Photographs Division: 56; © PresenterMedia: 4, 5, 19; © Shutterstock: 2, 12, 14, 25, 27, 28, 32, 34, 35, 41, 44, 48, 58, 62, 72, 74, 76, 77, 81; Courtesy of Anti-Racism & Cultural Diversity Office, University of Toronto www.antiracism.utoronto.ca: 70; Courtesy of Challenge of Change Project, Newry & Mourne District Council: 69; Courtesy of Independent Newspapers (Ireland) Limited: 68.

The author and publisher have made every effort to trace all copyright holders, but if any has been inadvertently overlooked we would be pleased to make the necessary arrangement at the first opportunity.

The article by Ailin Quinlan on pp. 30–1 is copyright Independent Newspapers Ireland, who we thank for permission to reproduce it here.

This book is typeset in Helvetica Neue 13/17.5 pt

The paper used in this book comes from the wood pulp of managed forests. For every tree felled, at least one tree is planted, thereby renewing natural resources.

All rights reserved. No part of this publication may be copied, reproduced or transmitted in any form or by any means, without permission of the publishers.

A CIP catalogue record for this book is available from the British Library.

5 4 3 2 1

Contents

Chapter 1 Listening and Speaking

Chapter outline 1
Introduction to communication 2
Key terms used in communication theory 4
One- and two-way communication 7
Types of listening required in different contexts 8
      Interpreting information 10
      Receiving information 11
Interpersonal communication 14
      Appropriate disclosure 16
      Oral communication skills 18

Chapter 2 Reading and Writing

Chapter outline 23
Reading skills 24
      Scanning, skimming and signposts 26
      Normal reading 27
      Close/critical reading 28
      Research and report writing 32

Writing skills 37
    Letter writing 41
        Personal letters 41
        Cover letters 42
Functional writing 44
    Curriculum vitae 45
    Incident reports 48
    Memos 50

Chapter 3 Non-Verbal and Visual Communication

Chapter outline 53
Perception 55
Barriers to communication in healthcare 58
    Hearing loss 59
    Sight loss 60
    Loss of speech 62
    Cognitive impairment 64
Visual communication 67
    Visual production 68

Chapter 4 Communications Technology

Chapter outline 71
The telephone 72
Computers 77
    Freedom of information 78

The internet 81
    Using the internet for research 84
Email 85

Appendix 1: Oral Presentation

Organising your presentation 89

Appendix 2: Assessment

Assessment portfolio 95
Grading 98

References 99

Chapter 1

Listening and Speaking

Chapter Outline

- Understand the key terms used in communication theory, such as sender, receiver, message, code, channel, communicate, noise, feedback and context, with particular reference to working life.

- Recognise the types of listening, such as understanding, interpreting, and receiving information, that are required in different contexts.

- Demonstrate a range of listening behaviours appropriate to the context, such as eye contact, facial expression, encouragement and control of own responses.

- Practise communication techniques relevant to different situations in work and leisure, such as conversations, interviews, formal presentations, message taking/giving and telephone dialogues.

Introduction to Communication

The process of communication has been described by McCabe and Timmins (2006) as both simple and complex. It is an essential skill required by healthcare assistants (HCAs) as it is at the core of all interactions we have with patients and indeed with other healthcare professionals. Care support staff spend more time at the client/service user's bedside than any other group of staff, and a large part of this time is spent communicating (Stonehouse 2014). Healthcare assistants who develop and reflect on their communication skills can make a significant difference in the care of clients/service users (Nazarko 2009). In this book we will examine the theoretical underpinnings of the concept of communication by defining the basic components of communication and exploring the influences which affect communication in the care setting.

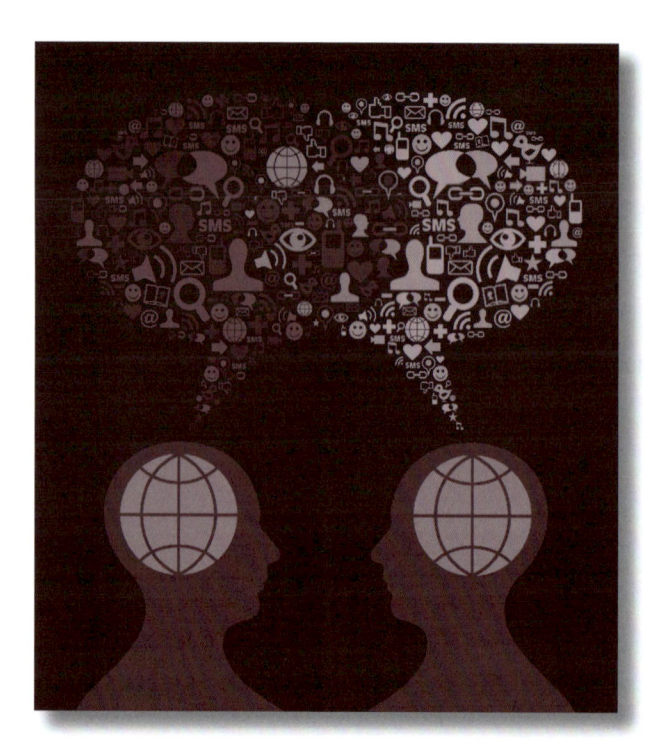

The word 'communicate' derives from the Latin word *communicare*, which means to share, impart or make common (Oxford Dictionaries 2014). The definition of communication is the *activity* of conveying meaningful information through a process of sending and receiving messages between two or more individuals to achieve a desired effect (Stephenson 2008). In order for effective communication to take place, Lewis (2014) argues that as well as sending information to the receiver, returning feedback to the sender is important to achieve clarity and avoid misunderstandings. All animals communicate in a variety of forms; for example, birds communicate by singing, gorillas by beating their chest and insects by performing a merry dance! In each form they are all imparting a message.

Why do we communicate? Dimbleby and Burton (2002) identify 12 purposes of communication:

1. Survival
2. Co-operation
3. Personal needs
4. Relationships
5. Persuasion
6. Power
7. Societal needs
8. Economy
9. Information
10. Making sense of the world

11. Decision making
12. Self-expression.

TASK

Choose three purposes of communication at work. Describe an example of how you communicate to achieve the appropriate outcome for each purpose.

For example, a nurse often has to persuade a patient of the needs and benefits of treatment in order to achieve the best possible outcome.

Key Terms Used in Communication Theory

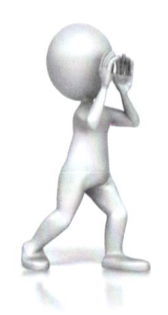

Sender: A sender is the person (or persons) who sends a message.

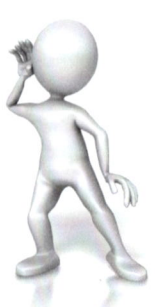

Receiver: A receiver is the person the message is sent to and who interprets the message. Some messages are literal and others have an implied meaning. For instance, is there ever an implied meaning to the question, 'Would you like to come in for a cup of coffee'?

Chapter 1 Listening and Speaking

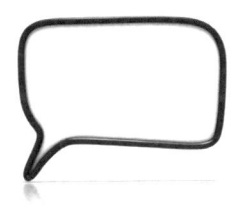

Message: This term has two aspects – the message the sender wants to communicate and the message the receiver interprets. People often think or say, 'Did I get that message across?'

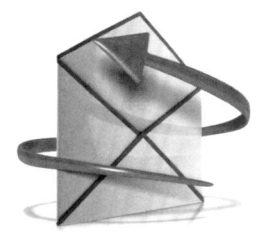

Code: Code is the way in which the sender (or source) wraps the message: the choice of language; the tone and body language that accompany a spoken message.

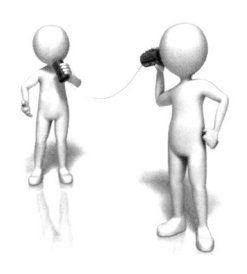

Channel: This is the way the message is transmitted, for example orally (face to face, by telephone), in actions or in writing (e.g. email).

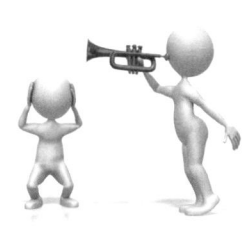

Noise: Noise means any kind of interference which interrupts or prevents the successful transmission of the message. It can be *physical* – pain can inhibit effective communication or the receiver may have a hearing, sight, speech or cognitive impairment; *emotional* – mistrust between the sender and receiver interfering with the message; *psychological* – a receiver who is tired and finding it difficult to take in a lengthy, complicated message; or *technological* – a fear of computers may prevent a person from using one to communicate.

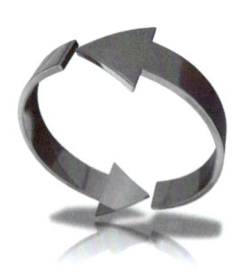

Feedback: If the process of communication is two-way and participative, the receiver will issue a response to the message. This response is called feedback. In doing this, the receiver then becomes the sender of a new message, creating a reciprocal process as the cycle begins again.

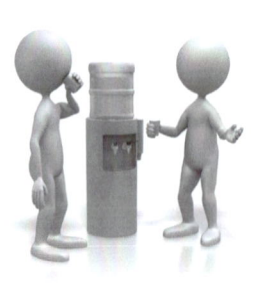

Context: This means the situation in which the communication takes place. It usually refers to time and place but may also include the people involved, for example at work in a hospital, or in a social venue like a pub.

TASK

Using the three examples you identified in the previous task, explain each in greater detail with reference to each of the key terms listed above.

One- and Two-Way Communication

Take part in this quick task in order to illustrate the pros and cons of one- and two-way communication. Then discuss the pros and cons of each method.

TASK

One-way communication: In the first part a volunteer will attempt to describe to the rest of the class, using words only, a specific shape given to them by the tutor. The sender will stand at the back of the room and the receivers will try to draw the shape based on the sender's descriptions. The sender should not see what the receivers are drawing.

Two-way communication: Now repeat the activity, except this time the sender stands at the front of the room facing the receivers, and the receivers may speak and ask questions.

THINK TANK

Take an example of a type of communication you have had at work in the past few days and analyse it under the following headings: message; your role as sender; the receiver's role (who was the receiver?); code; channel; context; feedback; noise. Was the communication successful? What could have been done to enhance the communication process?

Types of Listening Required in Different Contexts

Listening is as important if not more important than speaking, because without effective listening skills it is difficult to communicate with others. Listening is described by Nicklin and Kenworthy (2000) as a key element essential for effective helping. These authors propose that this skill is not as developed as we may suspect; often people are concentrating on their own problems, thoughts and feelings rather than listening to others. As the Chinese proverb says, 'Listen with your eyes, listen with your ears, listen with your heart and give undivided attention.'

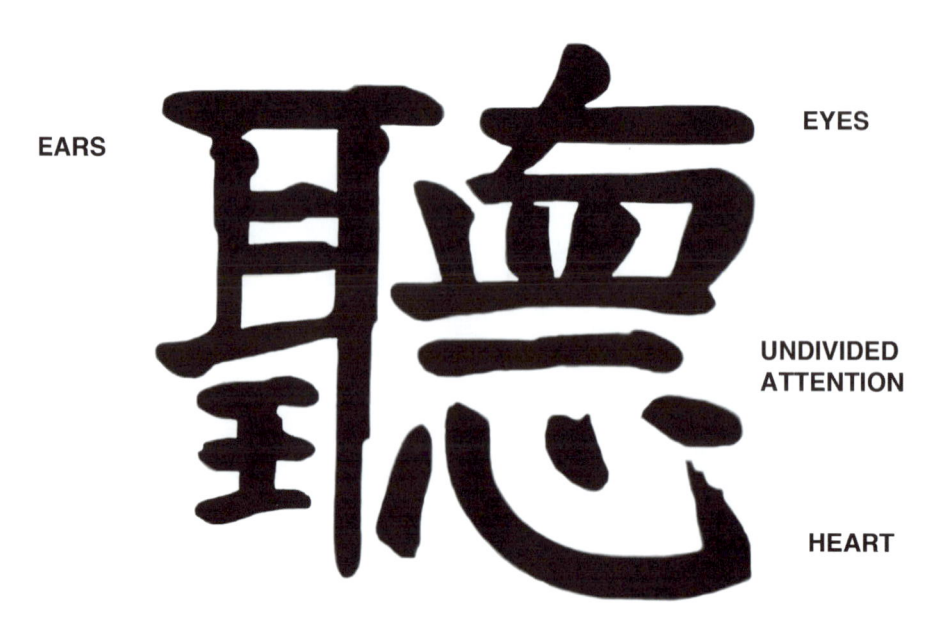

EARS

EYES

UNDIVIDED ATTENTION

HEART

The Chinese characters that make up the verb 'to listen' tell us something about this skill

Chapter 1 Listening and Speaking

Burnard and Gill (2008) state that listening refers to the process of hearing what the client is saying, encompassing not only the words that are being used, but also the non-verbal aspects of the encounter. This requires the carer to be fully present in the moment.

Julia Wood (2007: 184) describes five types of listening:

1. *Informational listening:* This involves listening for information such as facts, times, names and places. It is the most common type of listening that people do.

2. *Critical listening:* Critical listening entails making judgements and evaluations and forming opinions about a speaker's discourse. A teacher evaluates a student's oral presentation by listening critically for signs of careful preparation, structure, accurate information and good expression.

3. *Relational/empathetic listening:* An example of this type of listening is listening to a friend talk about their problems or worries. Relational listening often involves trying to understand how another person feels and interpreting the hidden signs that are behind the information that is heard.

4. *Listening for pleasure:* This is what a person does while playing a CD, or when they are at a concert, poetry reading or comedy show. Normally, this type of listening does not need too much concentration, unless the focus is on specifics like a lyric or a drum beat in a song.

5. *Listening to discriminate:* This is what a mechanic does when fine-tuning an engine and trying to detect a subtle

difference in sounds, or when parents decide if a child's crying is due to hunger, discomfort, a need for a nappy change or attention.

Interpreting Information

Selective listening: Hearing what one wants to hear. A person tends to pick and choose whom and what they want to listen to (Nida 1952). For the most part, this allows the person to give attention to people and subjects they are interested in or to focus on what can benefit them; the rest of the information is frequently ignored. For example, when a person is listening to an important message which needs to be passed on to someone else, they select the required information and omit the rest. Listening in an airport for announcements on flight delays, we listen only for our own flight and disregard all other information.

Active listening: This involves the skill of focusing on the central message of oral discourse by being able to actively resist distraction (Stonehouse 2014). A person shows the speaker that they are listening by giving verbal or non-verbal feedback, for example by saying 'Yes', 'Okay' or simply nodding. Verbal or non-verbal feedback has the effect of encouraging the speaker to communicate. It is like telling a joke – when everyone laughs, the speaker feels encouraged to tell another; if no one laughs, the speaker will usually stop. By giving feedback the listener is focused on the message, which itself helps listening and also gives encouragement to the speaker. This makes the communication more effective.

Interrupting: In general, interrupting a speaker is considered to be bad manners and can cause conflict. It can indicate that the listener has not been listening, is not interested or believes what they have to say is more important. However, there are occasions when interrupting is just part of the cut and thrust of the conversation. For example, during political debates on television and radio, members of the panel often say, 'If you would allow me to finish ...!' A person should always let someone finish their point before making their own contribution.

Responsive listening: Responsive listening shows the speaker that they have been not only listened to but also understood, and their feelings and circumstances acknowledged. The listener does not have to agree with what is said; and they have the option of saying either yes or no to a request. This type of listening allows for the possibility of further communication and helps to avoid conflict because it makes a distinction between acknowledgment and agreement.

Receiving Information

When faced with an hour-long talk or a full day's training, listening should not be a problem, but understanding and retaining information will be extremely difficult unless notes are taken. Most people are not capable of memorising all the information given during the course of an hour, so a written record that can be referred to later will help jog the memory.

Effective note taking: Start by heading the page with the date and subject. Try not to write down entire sentences: listen for a few minutes and then summarise what has been said, shortening everything, for example by using abbreviations for words and condensing sentences into keywords, phrases and headings. Leave out examples, anecdotes and irrelevant information; stick to the facts only. Flash cards can be very useful when revising to help stimulate your memory.

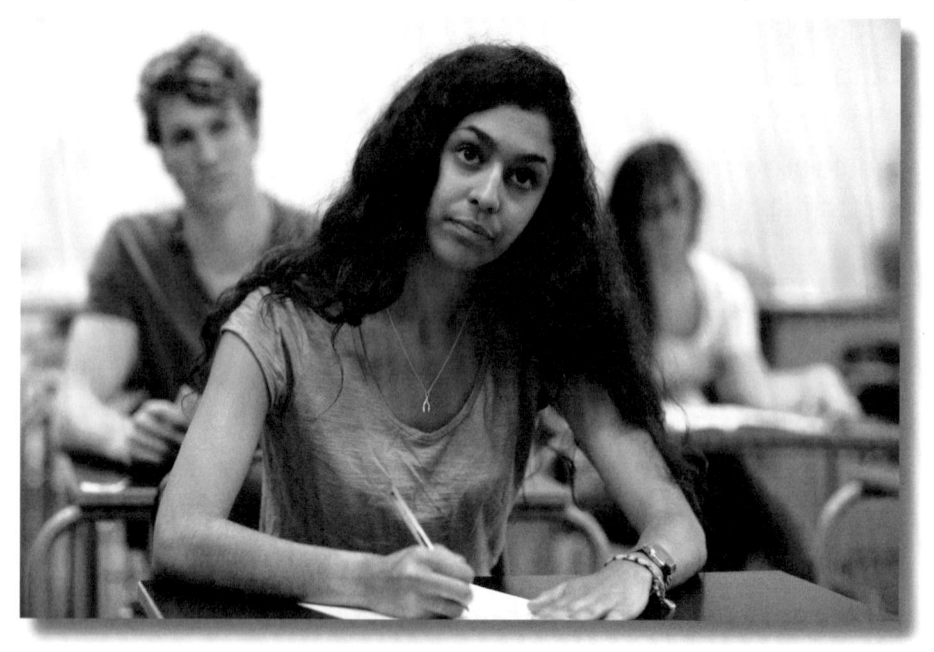

Here are some tips for effective listening:

1. Remove or resist distractions.
2. Make sure that you can hear properly.
3. Concentrate.
4. Focus on areas of interest and ask yourself, 'What am I getting out of this message?'
5. Be patient and listen to the full message before judging.
6. Give feedback.
7. Ask questions.

Chapter 1 Listening and Speaking

8. Keep an open mind and be objective.
9. Acknowledge the speaker and their emotional state.
10. Observe the speaker's body language and tone.
11. Avoid fidgeting, frowning and looking at your watch.

TASK

Watch the clips below on YouTube and take notes on what you think are good and poor listening skills.

- Bad listening skills: www.youtube.com/watch?v=U6b8Le3-yEc&feature=related
- *Everybody Loves Raymond* uses active listening: www.youtube.com/watch?v=4VOubVB4CTU

Demonstrate a range of listening behaviours appropriate to the context, such as eye contact, facial expression, encouragement and control of one's own responses.

Discuss a variety of examples of times at work when you find it difficult to listen effectively.

Watch the Managing Disclosure section of the *Open Your Eyes to Elder Abuse in the Community* video below as an example of good listening behaviours. Pay attention to how the community nurse communicates with Margaret and demonstrates effective and empathetic listening skills.

- www.youtube.com/watch?v=PkdoeSXj5fo&index=8&list=PL9BDE30D9532A0874

Interpersonal Communication

Interpersonal communication, or communication between people, is a key area of work for healthcare assistants because they are constantly interacting with clients/service users, and these interactions can involve matters of intimacy, privacy, stress, sickness and self-image. Therefore, the level of skill required in interpersonal communication is extremely high.

For example, an office worker might spend half of the day on the computer, a quarter of their time on the phone and perhaps an eighth on breaks and an eighth in face-to-face meetings, but they can still perform their job well even if their interpersonal skills are not highly developed. For healthcare, and specifically one-to-one care, the ratios are more than reversed, so interpersonal communication abilities have a massive impact on success as a healthcare assistant and a client/service user's success in recovery or daily living, overall self-image and emotional health.

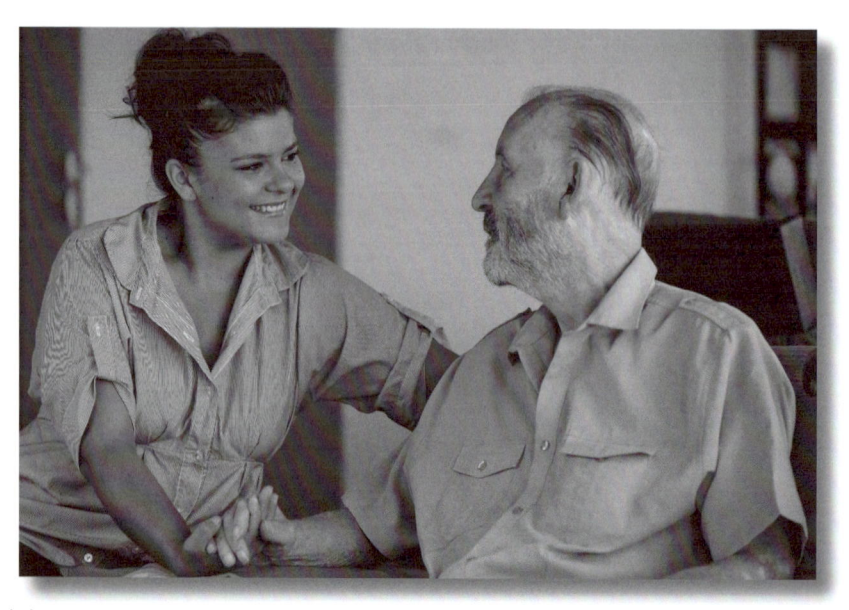

The passages that follow introduce some concepts and techniques which can help to create healthy interpersonal relationships and develop skills in this area.

Some key elements required to achieve good interpersonal communication include:

Non-judgemental attitude: A person who is non-judgemental can accept someone for who they are and what they are without imposing their own beliefs. Goldsborough (1970) states that being non-judgemental does not mean giving up personal beliefs or changing them to fit with what others think is morally right. What is at issue is whether practitioners are aware of their values and the importance they place on these values in the professional relationship they have with their patients.

Empathy: Empathy is the most critical ingredient in a helping relationship. It means the ability to understand and communicate an understanding of someone's experiences in a particular situation, as if it were your own situation (Kalisch 1971). It does not mean feeling sorry for someone (that is having sympathy), but rather actively supporting them.

Dual perspective: This means being able to recognise one's own values and a patient or client's values separately, i.e. being clear on whether one's actions are personally motivated or client-centred. Respecting and empowering clients/service users to make choices based on what *they* believe is right for them – as opposed to what the carer thinks is right for them – is key. According to the Health Information and Quality Authority (HIQA) (2009: Standard 17), each client/service user can exercise choice and control over his/her life and is encouraged and enabled to maximise independence in accordance with his/her wishes. Hence, care practices reflect a person-centred approach to care. The practitioner should encourage individuality and self-sufficiency, and promote the client/service user as an equal partner in his/her own care.

Climate: This is the understanding and assessment of timing; knowing the right time, place and moment to ask something of or state something to another person.

Self-disclosure: This means giving personal information to a client about one's own life or opinions. While self-disclosure does enhance relationships and develop communication, an understanding of boundaries is essential. Indeed, Ashmore and Banks (2002) state that it is not appropriate to disclose too much or too little in the carer–client/service user relationship, as either can inhibit the client/service user from dealing with their own concerns, hinder the development of therapeutic relationships and take time away from the patient.

Appropriate Disclosure

The healthcare assistant must be aware of certain boundaries and the potential impact of information shared when communicating with a client/service user. Carers are in a position of power and clients/service users are dependent on them and their ethical ability to do the right thing, regardless of personal opinion or preference. Therefore, healthcare assistants must always approach clients/service users objectively and keep subjective views aside. This responsibility is even more

Chapter 1 Listening and Speaking

important in any conversations or notes that are written down. That being said, in communication and relationship building, there is in general a need to share information in order to build trust and develop the relationship between the healthcare assistant and client/service user on a human level.

Look at the following table and consider in which context(s) it would be appropriate/inappropriate to disclose each type of information.

Contexts	Information
Job interview	Leisure activities
Family occasion	Career ambitions
Coffee with a close friend	Dreams
Meeting someone at a bus stop	Religious beliefs
On a first date	Personal achievements
An authority figure, e.g. your boss	Personal weaknesses
Work colleague	Confessions
Mother	Medical history
Client	Past experiences with drugs
Family members	Past experiences on holidays
New partner	Fantasies
Child	Thoughts on certain social groups
	A 'do not resuscitate' decision

Communications for Healthcare

> **TASK**
>
> Practise communication techniques relevant to different situations in work and leisure, such as conversations, interviews, formal presentations, message taking/giving and telephone dialogues.

Oral Communication Skills

Pitch and tone: Younger people have a naturally higher tone which deepens with age. The pitch and tone of a person's voice can communicate emotions such as whether they are sad, anxious, scared, happy or excited. Emotions can be communicated by a meek, low, slow voice or an accelerated, louder, gasping voice, which can run off into a pitch that is different from normal (a way of controlling this is to relax the muscles in the stomach, chest, shoulders and neck, and take controlled deep breaths with natural pauses in rhythm).

A monotonous tone is when the person does not change their tone or allow any emotion into their voice and delivery, which can be boring and unexciting to listen to. *Inflection* is the change of voice pitch depending on the message the person wants to convey. It can also add to the words being spoken by stressing particular words to communicate extra or implied meaning. This can enhance delivery and keep people interested; however, or 'how-ev-vaaaah' (Lauren from *The Catherine Tate Show*, see the link www.youtube.

com/watch?v=lzjD_7bRYmk), excessive inflection can communicate something entirely different.

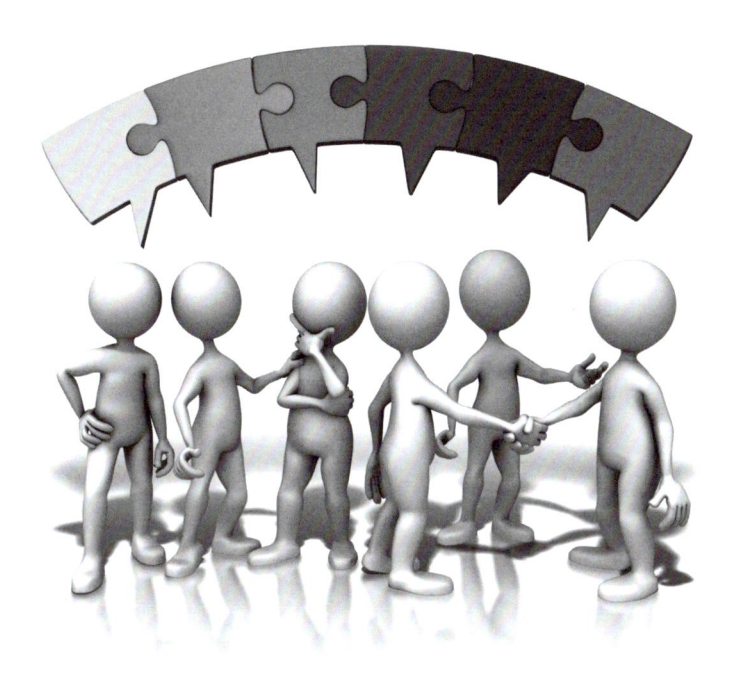

Volume: It is important to judge how loudly to speak. Over-loud voices can be off-putting and communicate the idea that the person is brash, boisterous and unable to listen; very quiet voices can suggest that a person is easily manipulated, meek or unassertive, or that they do not know what they are doing. If you are presenting to a group and people have to strain to hear you, they are likely to become irritated or lose interest. Hence, volume and control are extremely important when communicating with someone with any form of sensory disability.

Emphasis: We stress certain words to encourage the listener to receive a specific part of the information, for example 'Don't you *ever* do that again' or 'The train leaves from *platform number 3.*'

Pace/speed: Again, emotion can interfere with the ability to exert control in this area. If a person speaks too quickly or too slowly, they can easily lose their listeners and possibly miss out on something the listeners want to communicate to them. Self-awareness is key, as fast and slow speakers often do not recongnise these tendencies. During a presentation it is important for the speaker to check how they are speaking, take pauses and reiterate as well as checking that the audience has heard and understood them.

Articulation: This relates to, for example, contracting words and sentences, such as 'dontcha' and 'howya'. While this is fine in everyday use, it is not acceptable in more formal speech presentations. You do not need to change your accent, but you do need to challenge yourself to speak clearly and in a way that can be understood by everyone in your audience.

Presentation: When giving a spoken presentation it is important for the speaker, first, to be as comfortable as possible and, second, to present themselves in a way that does not detract from their presentation. Fidgeting, hesitating and using repetitive phrases can all do this. Staring at one person the whole time is not ideal as it excludes the rest of the audience. The speaker can take cues from the audience, which can help them gauge whether they are being understood, repeating themselves or doing well. Smiling and open body language can also help put the audience at ease, which in turn will put the speaker at ease.

TASK

Chose a task you undertake at work, such as at breakfast/dinner/bathing time, in which you find it difficult to communicate with a client/service user and write a description of this task. Make a list of the reasons why you have difficulty communicating; they could include, for example, fear, deafness or lack of understanding.

In groups of three, role play each of the tasks, with one member acting as the client/service user and the other giving feedback on communication skills.

In each of the settings listed below, identify a workplace example corresponding to the setting.

Settings: conversations, interviews, formal presentations, message taking/giving, and telephone dialogues.

Chapter 2

Reading and Writing

Chapter Outline

- Apply a reading approach appropriate to the purpose and the nature of the text to obtain an overview, identify key points, extract information, and undertake critical evaluation and in-depth analysis.

- Read critically, discriminately and with objectivity a range of media texts, including written, visual and broadcast texts.

- Plan and undertake research into a topic related to a vocational specialism, using a variety of sources, both primary (e.g. interviews and observations) and secondary (e.g. internet, media and libraries).

- Gather information from a range of written material, including technical/vocational, personal, literary, business and media communication material.

- Write clearly, confidently and expressively in a variety of forms relating to personal, creative, vocational and social needs.

- Follow the conventions of writing for a specific purpose, including writing letters, reports and memoranda.

- Use with confidence the vocabulary and language conventions relevant to a specific area of work.

- Observe the current conventions of written English usage (such as spelling, punctuation and syntax) in accordance with purpose.

- Draft, edit and proofread written documents.

Reading Skills

TASK

Make a list of all of the types of material you have read over the past 24 hours. Which is the most common type of reading material for you? Is this similar to the rest of the group? Discuss.

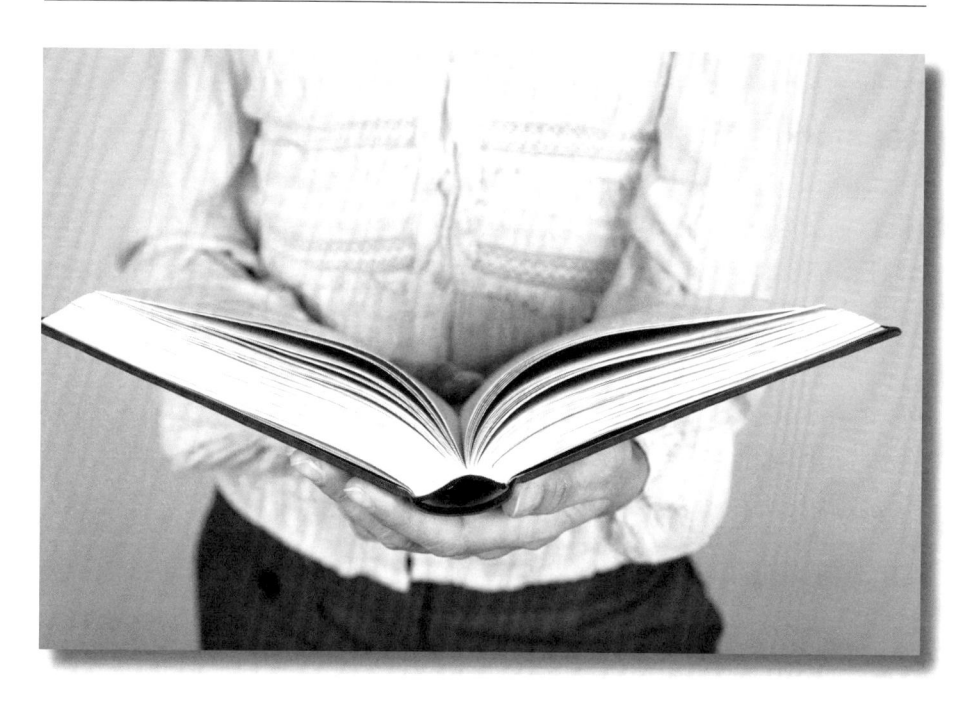

As a student on any healthcare course you will be required to read literature; hence, active reading is a skill you will be required to develop. Take a look at the reading list for your course and you will see that academic tutors place great value on reading. In fact, active reading is essential for success in your course. For your assessment you may be asked to select and write a short report on a piece of media or article related to healthcare. This written report can be based on an article, a leaflet, advertisement, poster, radio or television advertisement or an internet source. Just remember that you need to produce the source of the report as part of the assessment. In order to prepare the report you need to be able to enhance your technical reading skills.

Scanning, Skimming and Signposts

Scanning: This is reading that is purpose-driven for information that we specifically need, such as using dictionaries and timetables; we skip most of the information, and seek out keywords of interest to us. For instance, have you ever skimmed through a newspaper article looking for your own name and then closely read the context surrounding your name? Scanning is useful in building information for a research project, allowing the reader to pick out relevant sections from a variety of sources.

Skimming: This means swiftly glancing across the text to get an idea of the general theme or gist of the content. The reader skips over the parts that are not relevant to their needs, but if they find something relevant, they can go back and read a section more closely. Skimming is much like scanning except that the reader is not looking for a particular reference but trying to understand the main theme of the piece. When buying a new book, people sometimes skim through the first few pages to see if they like the book or whether they should put it back on the shelf.

This YouTube video on skimming and scanning might be useful: www.youtube.com/watch?v=GIHt8kHMUtc

Signposts: These are headings, sub-headings and headlines. Signposts help the reader to organise reading and understand the content. This also helps the writer to organise their material and stay focused on the topic.

Chapter 2 Reading and Writing

> **TASK**
>
> Take a look at a magazine and identify the various signposts. See how many you can pick out on one page.

Normal Reading

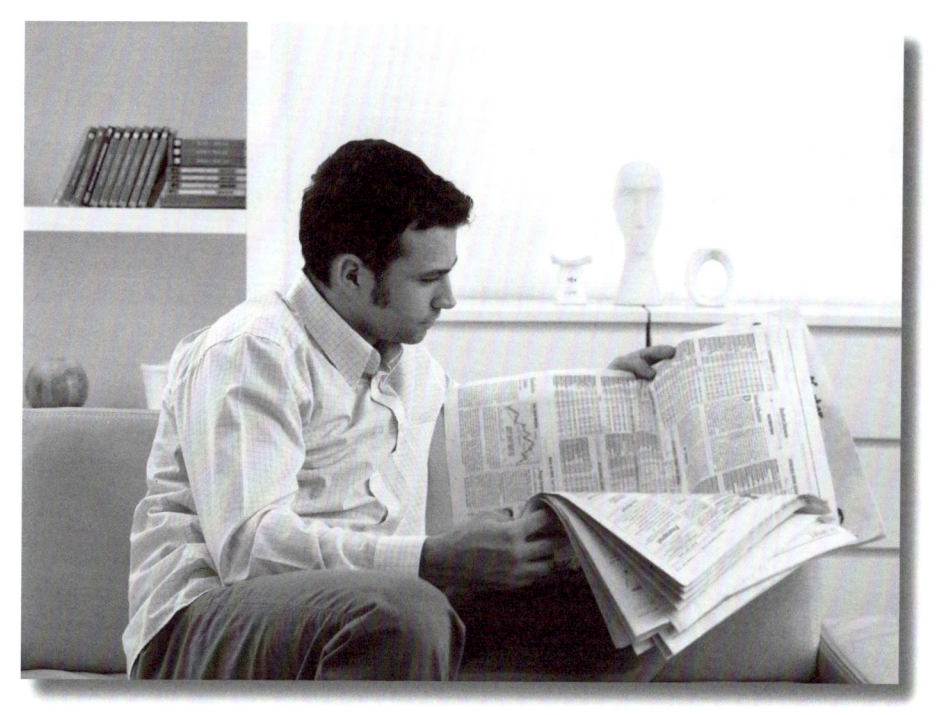

Normal reading means reading at a moderate speed, for example when reading novels, letters, newspaper articles and magazines. A lack of speed is considered to be a major reading problem as it is found that with increased speed comes better understanding. The average person reads at about 250 words per minute with a comprehension rate of about 60 per cent

(Cowen *et al.* 2009). If a person reads one word at a time, they can often lose concentration and forget what has just been read; this sometimes results in daydreaming, or getting bogged down in minute details.

Fixations are natural pauses that occur while reading when our eyes are drawn to a particular part of a passage. The number of words we focus on during a fixation is called our recognition span.

Close/Critical Reading

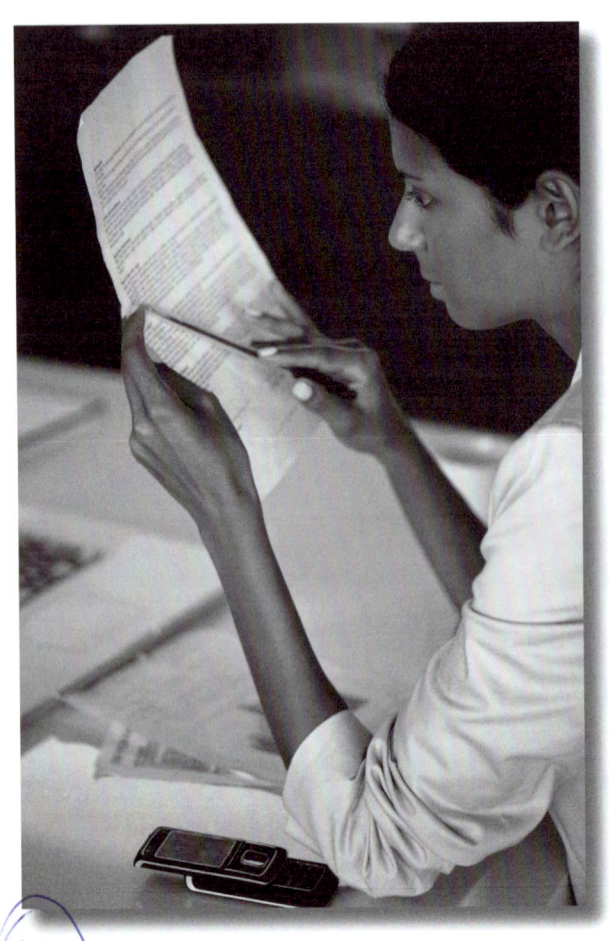

This is a slow and intensive method of reading. The text may be demanding or the information more important than normal, for example a lease or contract, exam instructions or material for exam study. It is very difficult to sustain this type of reading, so it should be done in no more than 40-minute segments.

Critical reading is a dynamic skill and one that you need to practise. Here are some tips for close or critical reading:

1. Note down information that you already know.
2. Note down information that is interesting and relevant.
3. Break long sentences into smaller chunks.
4. Write down, underline or highlight difficult words and passages.
5. Look up any unfamiliar words in a dictionary.
6. After reading, try to remember the main points of what you have read. Write them down.
7. Go over the passage once more in case you have missed anything.
8. After you have read the passage try to recall in your own words what it said.

TASK

Read the article on the next page using the following process: (a) scan it first for words that you do not understand and underline them; (b) look up these words in the dictionary or consult your tutor; (c) skim the article to grasp the main theme; (d) read the whole article again normally to understand it more fully; and (e) read it closely to discover any hidden meanings or sections open to interpretation.

Communications for Healthcare

Post-cancer fatigue doesn't have to be endured forever

Many patients find that fatigue is one of the most distressing symptoms following cancer

Ailin Quinlan

YOU'VE endured the shock of a cancer diagnosis, and suffered the energy-draining treatment – now, surely you can expect to get your life back. But instead you cannot shake off the debilitating cloud of fatigue that has descended upon you.

Between 70 per cent and 99 per cent of chemotherapy and radiotherapy patients report fatigue during and after treatment, according to research, while about a third of disease-free cancer survivors report persistent fatigue between six months and 10 years after completing treatment.

Meanwhile, more than 50 per cent of women with breast cancer struggle with insomnia following treatment and this can feed cancer-related fatigue.

This fatigue is described by many patients as the most distressing of all symptoms following cancer – more so, says Dr Sonya Collier, than pain and depression. But now there's help.

A new manual and accompanying DVD offers hope to sufferers.

Manual

Described as 'therapy in a book' by Dr Collier, principal clinical psychologist in the Psychological Medicine Service at St James's Hospital, the manual has been written by Collier in conjunction with Dr Anne Marie O'Dwyer, consultant psychiatrist in the Psychological Medicine Service at St James's.

'We noticed that many of the patients we saw following cancer treatment were struggling with fatigue,' says Collier.

'That fatigue was having a serious impact on the quality of their lives. They didn't realise what it was or how to cope with it, and many people believed it was something they just had to endure.'

Cancer-related fatigue, she explains, is very different from normal fatigue.

'It's overwhelming and is not relieved by rest. It impacts on the patient's normal day-to-day activities and causes a lot of emotional distress – some people may not feel able to get out of bed in the morning or they may be sleeping a lot during the day.'

People who tend to be most badly affected are those who have had both radiotherapy and chemotherapy.

'It's thought to be almost normal in people who have had both types of treatment. For many patients the fatigue will improve over time, for some it will persist long term.'

These are the people at whom the 200-page *Understanding and Managing Persistent Cancer-Related Fatigue* and its accompanying DVD are specifically aimed, she says.

'The manual is written for people whose fatigue has persisted for at least six months.'

The book, says Collier, can help people tackle some of the factors that can feed into cancer-related fatigue: sleep problems, anxiety, low mood and lack of exercise.

'These are common factors that can cause cancer-related fatigue in patients. A lot of patients think their cancer fatigue is due solely to chemotherapy or radiotherapy or side effects and that can be true during and immediately after treatment.'

Cycle

Psychological factors can play a role, and the book, she says, shows how 'unhelpful thinking and action can feed into a vicious cycle'.

Its aim, says Collier simply, is to help people break that vicious cycle.

Launched recently at St James's Hospital, the manual is crammed with patient stories, helpful information and user-friendly charts, as well as illustrations tackling issues such as inactivity, low mood, sleep problems, worry and reclaiming life after cancer.

The accompanying DVD features well-known personalities such as Kathryn Thomas, Pat Kenny, Rachel Allen, Charlie Bird, Miriam O'Callaghan, Eddie Hobbs, Diarmuid Gavin and Dermot Earley to explain the different issues.

■ Patients of St James's Hospital will get the manual and DVD free through the hospital, while the programme is also to be distributed to the other centres of excellence in Cork, Limerick, Dublin, Galway and Waterford.

Irish Independent
24 October 2011

Communications for Healthcare

TASK

The more we read, the better we become at writing. Discuss.

Research and Report Writing

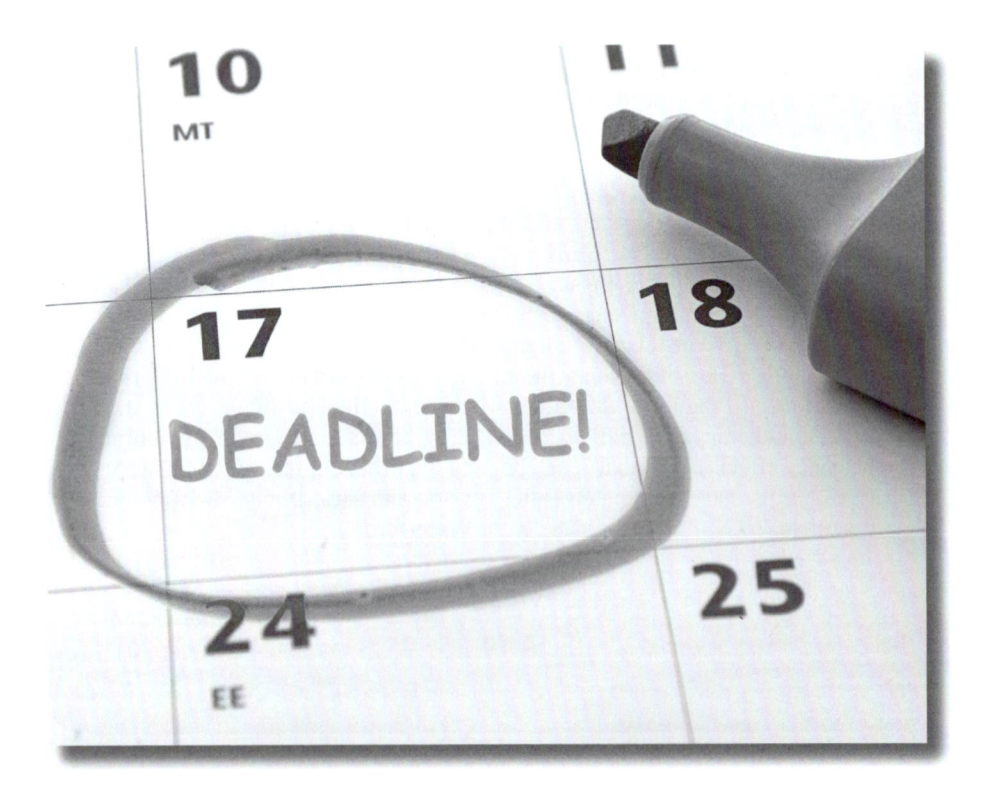

Preparation: First up, make a note of the deadline! If you miss the deadline, the assignment may not be marked or you may incur a penalty. Work out how much time you have to write the assignment, bearing in mind the time you need to plan, word process, proofread and polish. Organisational aspects in the final stage almost always take longer than allowed for; these include referencing, spell check, page numbering and layout of images and/or tables. Set aside specific times during the week as 'assignment time', in much the same way as if you were planning to go to the gym or attending a social event. Part of putting together a report is being organised and if you do a little every week for the three weeks of this course, or whatever the duration of the module, you will have more chance of success than if you cram it all into the last few days at the end.

Tips for choosing a topic:

1. Choose a topic that you are interested in.
2. Check if it is easy to research.
3. Ensure that it is work related.
4. Be able to write a specific title.

Research: Researching a topic can involve two types of research: *primary research*, which is new research carried out by the researcher, e.g. interviews, questionnaires or experimentation; and *secondary research*, which is reading previously written articles/research carried out by others and referencing that information to create your own report.

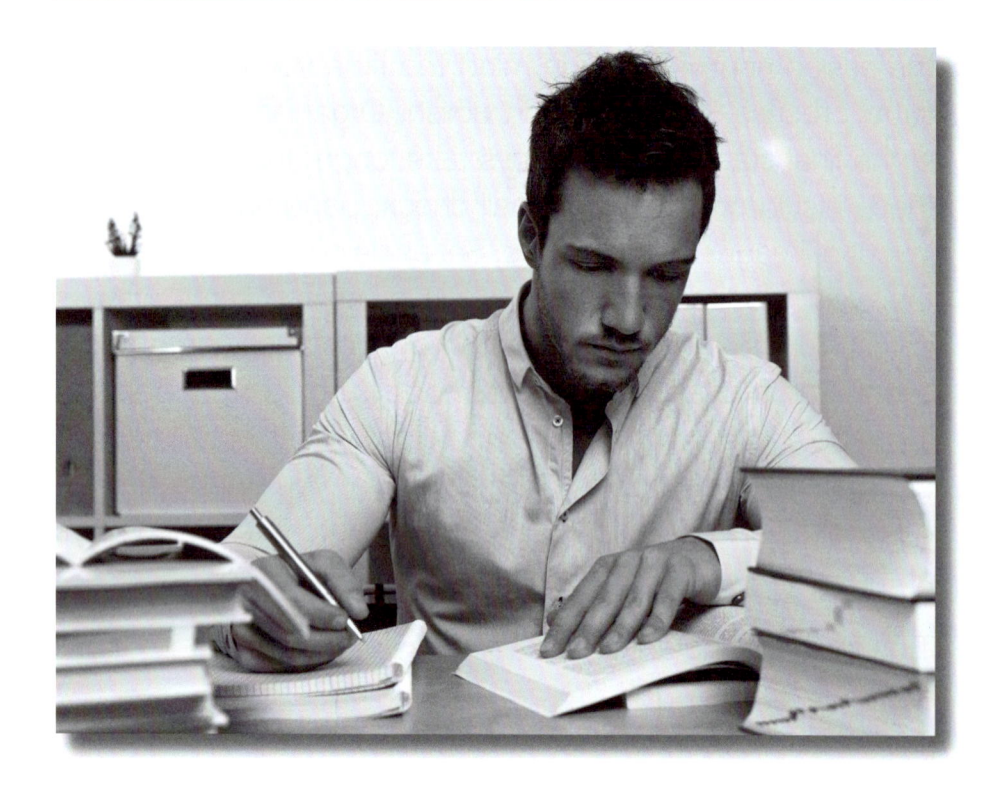

Secondary research is the most common and it is the type of research used for assignments on this course. Sources of information include the internet, newspapers, magazines, other publications, encyclopaedias and libraries. Carrying out extensive research will improve the report, but be careful to leave enough time after researching to structure and write the report.

Format: The report comprises three main parts. The *introduction* explains the purpose of the report, the area of interest and how it has been researched. The *main body*, written as a series of sections or paragraphs, informs the reader of all the relevant areas in detail. Sub-headings or chapter titles may be added to each of these sections. Once the area of interest has been researched, the sub-headings should be mapped as shown in the diagram on page 39. The *conclusion*, which comes at the end of the report, summarises the main findings or themes discovered from the research. Future research topics and how they will progress your own report can be included. A mind map or concept map can help early on when brainstorming what should be covered in your assignment (Kneale and Santy 2000).

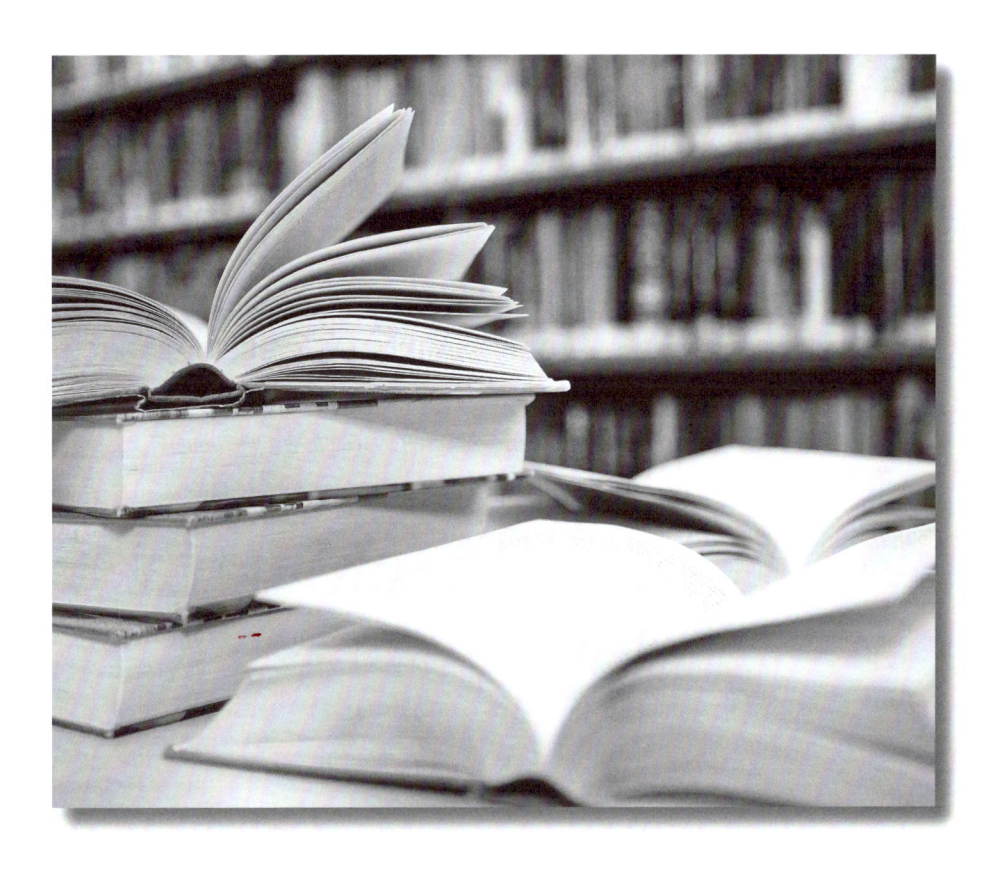

References: When using secondary research as a main method of finding information about a research topic, the authors of articles and books used should be credited. This can be done in a few ways. Quotations are used when you want to use word-for-word excerpts from a particular source. Use double quotation marks (" ") and keep the quotation as short as possible, using only the information that is absolutely relevant. At the end of the quotation include the author's name and the year in which the piece was written.

If you want to use a general idea expressed in a piece of secondary research but describe it in your own words, simply put the author's name and year of writing in brackets at the end of the section or begin the description in this way: 'In the *Sunday Independent* (May 2010) Brendan O'Connor wrote ...'

The references should be listed in greater detail after the conclusion of the report, so that the reader can, if they want, find and read an original article. A reference should include the author's name, book (or article) title, year and place of publication, journal title (for articles), name of publisher, and page numbers of relevant text.

For more information on using the Harvard referencing system, which is the most common referencing system used in nursing and healthcare assignments, download the *School of Nursing and Midwifery Harvard Referencing Guide* under the Training Materials section at: www.tcd.ie/Library/support/subjects/nursing-midwifery/.

Chapter 2 Reading and Writing

TASK

Media treatment of healthcare issues

This is an activity to do at home.

1. Using a variety of sources, e.g. newspapers, magazines and the internet, identify several healthcare-related news items.
2. Read each item using the method described earlier under the task at Close/Critical Reading.
3. Compare and contrast each item in terms of the general theme, writing style and key words used.
4. Make some short notes.

Use this opportunity to identify a topic that you might be particularly interested in; then you can use this theme for your report and presentation.

Writing Skills

TASK

List as many different forms of writing as you can in one minute.

All the writing methods identified in this section generally involve the same preparation before being published:

1. *Purpose/intention:* What do you want to achieve? What effect do you want to have on the reader?
2. *Topic:* What is the piece of writing going to be about?
3. *Form:* In what way will the piece of writing be written?
4. *Language:* This includes thinking about the kinds of words that will be used to create the style. Are slang words or abbreviations appropriate, for instance?
5. *Personal style:* Ensure that any commonly used words or expressions complement the form and purpose. If your assignment is reflective it is appropriate to write in the first person; otherwise generally refer to yourself as 'the writer'.
6. *Punctuation and grammar:* Double-check and proofread to make sure that punctuation and grammar are correct.

Once the preparation is complete the piece should be completed in this order:

Plan/rough notes/map: This is a brainstorming session and forms the backbone of the writing. Identify key points and important topics; then put them in an order that is appropriate and will help the piece flow. Sub-topics may also be included. Now, brainstorm a topic of interest in healthcare using the diagram on the next page.

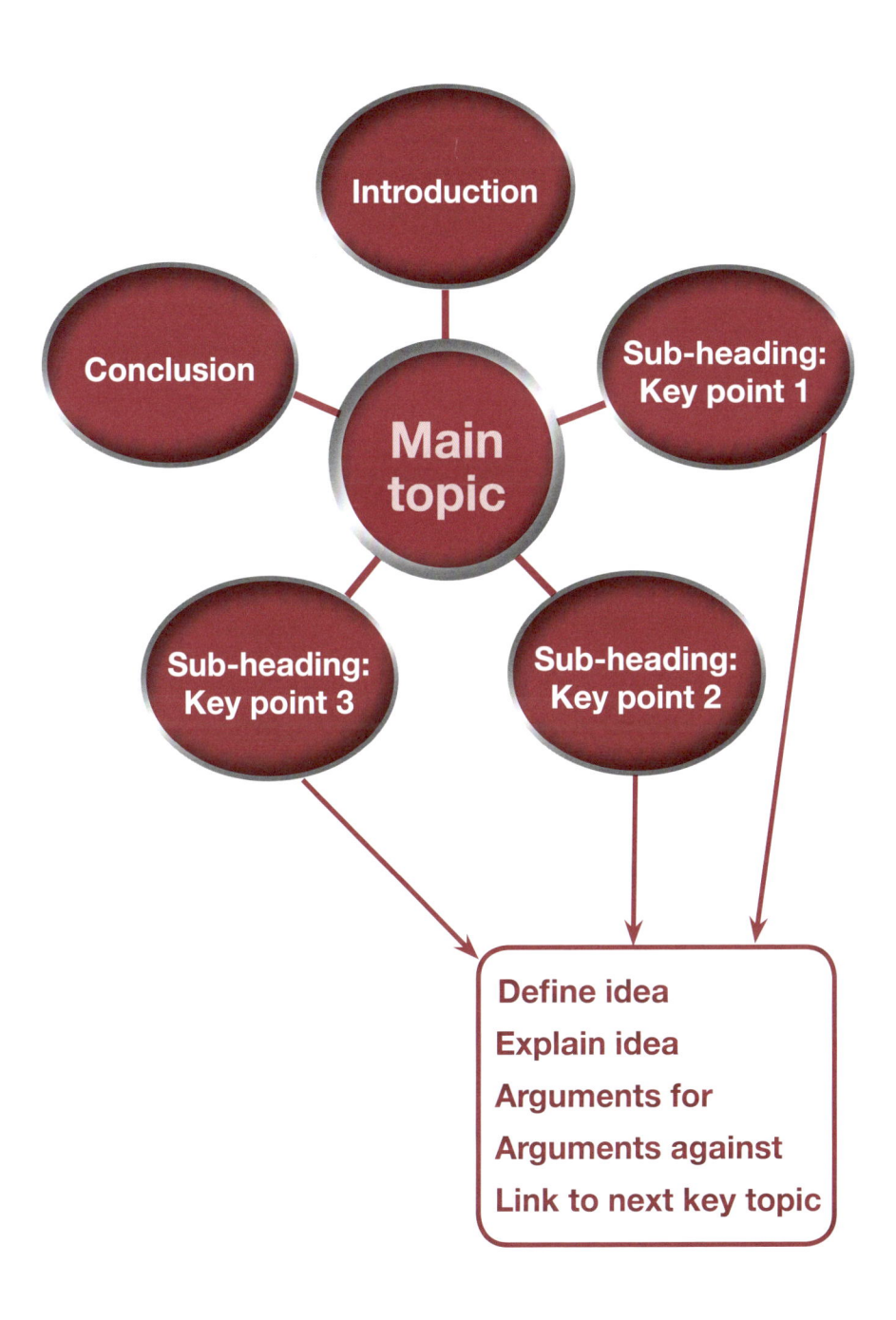

- Introduction
- Conclusion
- Main topic
- Sub-heading: Key point 1
- Sub-heading: Key point 2
- Sub-heading: Key point 3

- Define idea
- Explain idea
- Arguments for
- Arguments against
- Link to next key topic

Draft: The draft involves writing in more detail about each area, attempting to convey a message or meaning in each section. It is best to write in a style that flows freely and is comfortable for you. In fact, it is far better to free write your first draft. Don't limit yourself with rules; just write your thoughts as they come to you. You can restructure your drafts later. Many novice students are tempted to copy and paste information from the internet and claim it as their original work. This is plagiarism, and there are consequences for plagiarising others' work. If you write your assignment in your own words and later add references, you are not plagiarising. Reread quickly what you have just written, but do not dwell too much – carry on getting all of the ideas, thoughts and research down on paper. Then you can start the editing process.

Redraft/edit: This stage involves rereading carefully what has been written and examining its meaning. Ask yourself if what has been written conveys the message you want to communicate to the reader. If there are sections you are unhappy with, reword them until you are satisfied or leave them out entirely. Although it may feel a little foolish, read your work aloud; if you do this you are far more likely to notice any errors in your sentence structure, grammar and spellings.

Proofread: It is wise to get someone else to proofread your work – they may see mistakes you have not noticed.

Letter Writing

Personal Letters

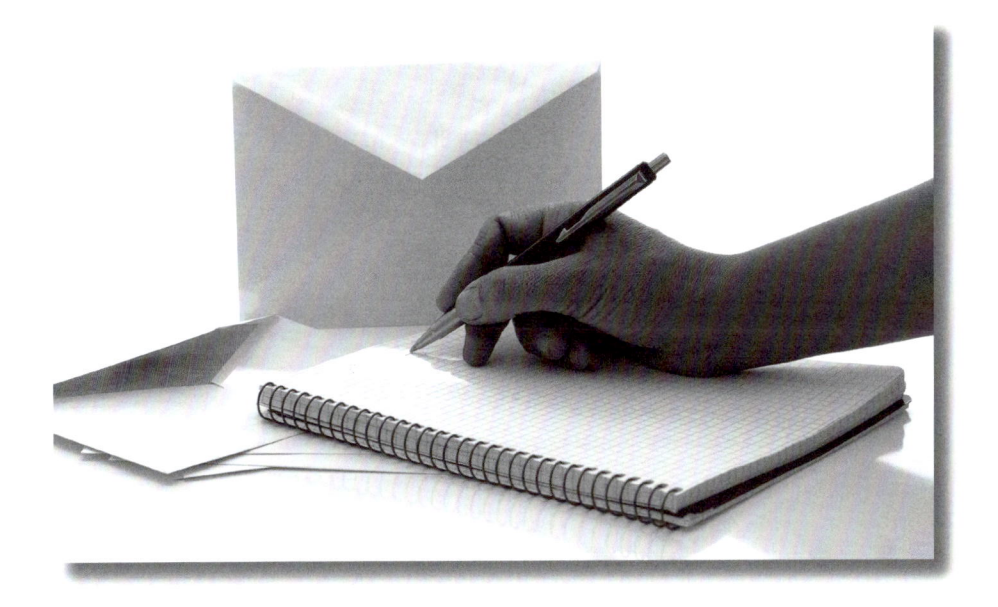

With the development of communications technology, such as email and text messaging, writing and posting personal letters is much less common nowadays. Nevertheless, sending a personal letter will resonate with the receiver as a letter will have more of an impact and will appear thoughtful. People often keep letters they have received because they have sentimental value. Personal writing, such as writing a letter to a friend, is informal, but there is a simple structure and method to putting the message on paper:

1. The sender's address should go on the top right-hand corner of the page.
2. The date goes below the sender's address.

3. The salutation (greeting, e.g. 'Dear John') begins below the date but on the left-hand side of the page.

4. Indent the first line of each paragraph.

5. Finishing the letter is familiar and informal, for example 'Lots of love', 'All the best' or 'Yours' are typical, depending on your relationship with the receiver.

> **TASK**
>
> Structure a personal letter using the above steps.

Other types of personal writing include a poem you have written yourself, a blog about a topic you are interested in, or a short story.

Cover Letters

A cover letter is a formal letter. For example, a cover letter accompanies a curriculum vitae (CV) to explain a person's motivation in applying for a job. In many cases the cover letter is sent via email with the CV attached, but in some cases the prospective employer may specify that the application must be made by post and/or the cover letter handwritten. It is important to follow instructions!

The structure and content of the cover letter may be a deciding factor when it comes to being called for interview. Follow the method described below:

Header: On the top right-hand side of the page put your address, telephone number, email address and the date below it. On the next line down from this but on the left-hand side of the page, put the name of the person in charge of the applications, their title role and the company address. Begin the body of the letter with 'Dear Mr/Mrs/Ms'.

First paragraph: Be precise about the position for which you are applying and include where you read/heard about it.

Second paragraph: Refer to your CV and add anything of particular relevance to the position for which you are applying.

Third paragraph: Round off with a statement of expected outcome, e.g. 'I look forward to hearing from you in response to my application.'

Finish: Appropriate closings include 'Yours sincerely' or 'Regards'. Below this sign the letter and print your name underneath the signature.

Before writing, find out the details of the position for which you are applying. If possible, find out the name of the person to whom you should apply and address the letter to that person by name. Find out what they are looking for and sell yourself accordingly. Be sincere, truthful and quietly confident. Never send original papers of references or certificates; always send copies. Keep copies of all the letters you send.

Communications for Healthcare

TASK

Write a cover letter in response to an advertisement in the local newspaper, which is seeking a healthcare assistant to work in a facility in which you already work or in the type of facility in which you would like to work, e.g. hospital, nursing home or homecare. Follow the method described above.

Functional Writing

There are three types of functional writing relevant to communications for healthcare: the curriculum vitae, incident reports and memos.

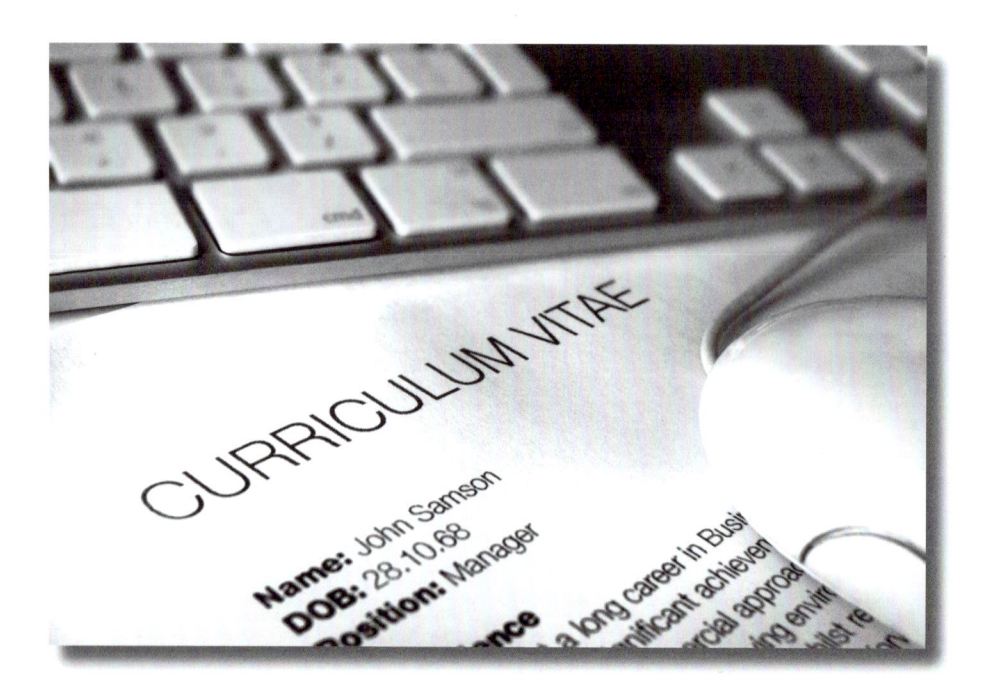

Curriculum Vitae

Curriculum vitae (CV) means 'course of life' in Latin. This document is intended to give a brief account of a person's life to date. It should be word-processed, neatly presented and well laid out, with the most important and relevant information appearing first. There are many computer programs available to help structure a CV and, even easier, most jobsites have templates to help job seekers get started. All the following information should be included in the CV:

1. *Personal details:* Name, address, phone number and email address.

2. *Education and qualifications:* The standard is for these to be listed in reverse chronological order (most recent first), with dates, courses, subjects, prizes/awards, work placements, detail of equipment used (if relevant), and final project/dissertation.

3. *Work experience/employment history:* These should also be listed in reverse chronological order, with dates, names of employers, job titles and experience acquired.

4. *Additional information:* Other skills and abilities such as computer or language proficiency and achievements such as completing a marathon or organising a fundraising event.

5. *Interests and activities:* These include membership of clubs, societies, organisations and positions of responsibility.

Communications for Healthcare

6. *Referees:* These can include previous employers/teachers. Always ask your referees for permission before you add them to your CV. You can state that references are available on request.

TASK

Use the following template to help you create your CV.

CV Template

Name

Address

Telephone (home)/mobile

E-mail

Personal Profile

Summary about what you have done (qualifications, relevant experience etc.); the skills you have to offer

Education and Qualifications

Date   University/college, course, qualification (grade or predicted grade)

	Subject
	Modules studied, dissertation
Date	Secondary school/college

Work Experience (most recent first)

Date	Company name, job title
	Main responsibilities
	Skills gained (e.g. communication, team work, interpersonal, problem solving)

Additional Information (skills and abilities)

Languages

IT

Other relevant skills

Interests and Activities

Do not just supply a list – try to make each interest/activity relevant to what the employer is looking for. For example: 'Travelling around Europe and meeting a variety of people helped to develop my communication skills.'

References

Available on request

Communications for Healthcare

Incident Reports

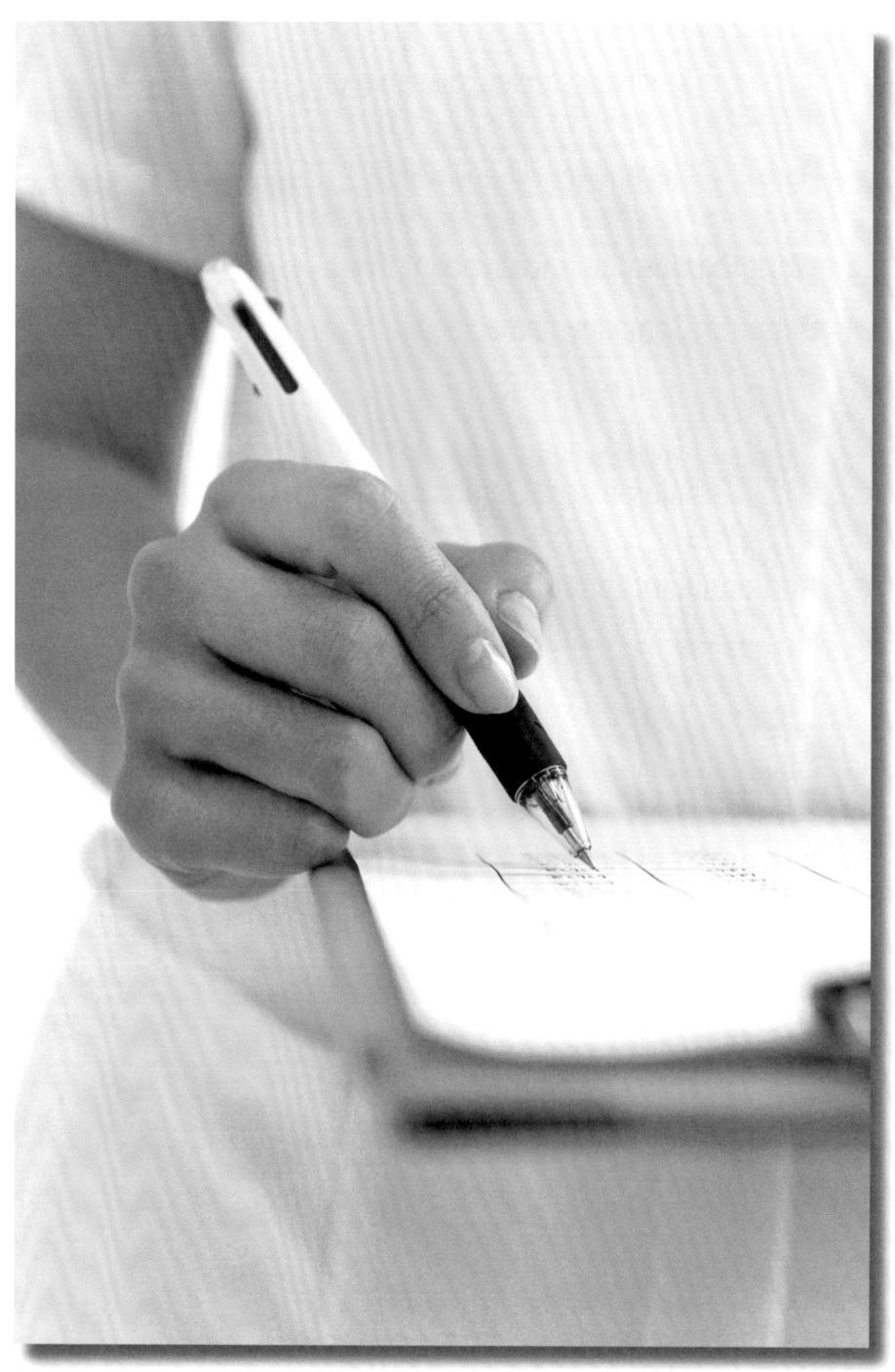

Every year, over a thousand injuries are reported to the Health and Safety Authority (HSA) by the health and social work sector (HSA 2014). This accounts for nearly 20% of all workplace injuries reported to the HSA each year. There are three main accident triggers in the healthcare sector:

1. Manual handling (patient handling and handling of inanimate loads)
2. Slips, trips and falls (on the level)
3. Work-related shock, fright and violence.

See more at:

www.hsa.ie/eng/Your_Industry/Healthcare_Sector/Healthcare_Illness_and_Injury_Statistics/#sthash.YYpdCavX.dpuf.

As is mandatory in any healthcare setting, if there is an incident in which a staff member/client/other person is harmed, an accident report must be completed by all who witnessed the accident. The accident report enables the event to be revisited should there need to be a change of treatment or if litigation is initiated. The report should be completed immediately or as soon as possible after the incident has occurred. An incident report should also be carried out if a hazard has been identified or if there has been a potentially dangerous event at work, even if no one was injured. The forms are created by the employer and should be filled out according to the instructions on the form.

Communications for Healthcare

> **TASK**
>
> Discuss the pros and cons of using accident and incident report forms to detail incidents in the healthcare setting.

Memos

A memo (shortened from the word memorandum) is a short message used internally in organisations to convey or request information, confirm spoken information or give instructions. The word memorandum comes from the Latin word meaning 'something to be remembered'. Many companies have their own standardised memo forms. A range of items can be included on a memo but generally the most important are the sender, the recipient, the date and the subject matter.

Memo

To:

From:

Date:

Re.:

Body text here…

Chapter 3

Non-Verbal and Visual Communication

Chapter Outline

- Recognise the role of perception in the communication process and the factors that affect it, such as sensory variation, stereotyping and prejudice.

- Demonstrate an awareness of the ways in which we communicate non-verbally through gesture, posture, appearance, eye and physical contact, facial expression, proximity and orientation.

- Demonstrate appropriate non-verbal communication in a range of settings, including one-to-one, group, formal and informal.

- Construct and interpret visual aids and/or images.

Communications for Healthcare

TASK

Carry out a two-way conversation without speaking and see if you can communicate the messages below.

Person A	Person B
Hello	Hello
Are you all right?	I'm all right. And you?
So so!	What time is it?
I don't know	Can you give me some money?
No	Please
No!	I'm hungry
I don't have any money	I'm cold
Look over there	What? Where? I don't see anything
It doesn't matter	Goodbye
Goodbye	

Perception

Perception is the ability a person has to take in the whole picture around them with all five senses. According to Swann (2009), perception is how the brain sifts through the multitude of information it receives and makes sense of this information. Children can do this accurately before they learn to speak. People often rely on perception to give them cues about their surroundings, dangers and people they come into contact with. An adult's perception of things can be how they select, organise and interpret their experiences. However, perception can be misleading, for example train tracks appear to get narrower the further away they are; a siren sounds different when it passes than when it is behind us. So although perception is important in lots of ways, it can also be inaccurate. Furthermore, as individuals we perceive the same circumstances differently. Thus perception, although a tool for forming an opinion, can only ever be a part of the whole picture. See the drawing on the next page and discuss what you perceive.

Communications for Healthcare

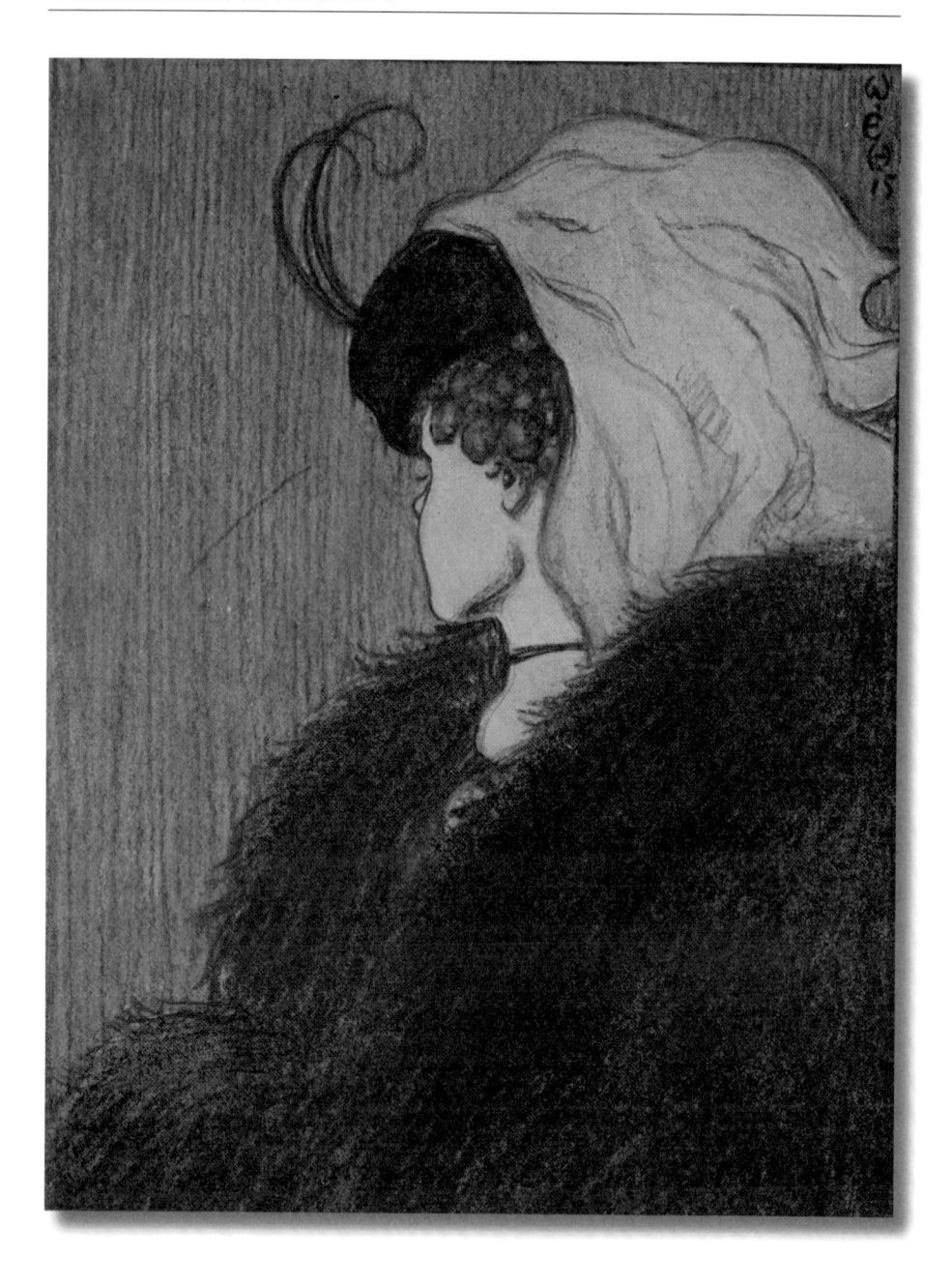

Selection is the process by which a person filters the information that they perceive. Often, this is how people with the same experience remember different things or remember things differently. Perception can be based on other experiences the person has had, or listening to or seeing the experiences of others. As children we learn a lot through **modelling**: children tend to copy behaviours and opinions they have been exposed to by adults or older children. Bandura (1977) claimed that how much the observer learns from an experience depends on their incentive and motivation to learn. All of these things form a person's beliefs and reactions to the people, places and things they meet and experience. When faced with a situation or a particular person, an individual may recall any previous experience or information they have been told in order to prepare themselves; and they often form opinions and judgements based purely on this as opposed to the reality of the new experience. It is very important to be aware of this, as people often bring **bias and discrimination** to those they meet or to new situations.

People are products of their environments and societies; they grow up and live in communities or cultures which have certain values, rituals and rules, and most tend to be moulded and shaped by these rules. **Stereotyping** involves judging those who are strangers or judging an entire group based on an experience with one member of that group. In today's mobile society and transient population it is not enough to be aware only of your own culture. **Culture** and **cultural norms** are described as a way of life which includes knowledge, beliefs, morals, laws, customs and other attributes acquired by a person as a member of society (Burnard and Gill 2008), and cultures vary greatly throughout the world, which often leads to misinterpretation or **prejudice** when one culture is perceived to be valued as more 'correct'.

It is expected that the healthcare assistant will meet many different types of clients/service users from various cultural backgrounds. Each client/service user has the right to their own thoughts and opinions. They also have the right to the same care as someone else who might fit better with 'our own' ideas on how to live life or behave. Whether or not the healthcare assistant agrees with someone's choices on a personal level, they need to be aware of the ways they might communicate their own beliefs verbally or non-verbally to others.

Barriers to Communication in Healthcare

There are a number of possible barriers to communicating with clients/service users receiving healthcare. However, there are ways in which the healthcare assistant can learn to communicate effectively.

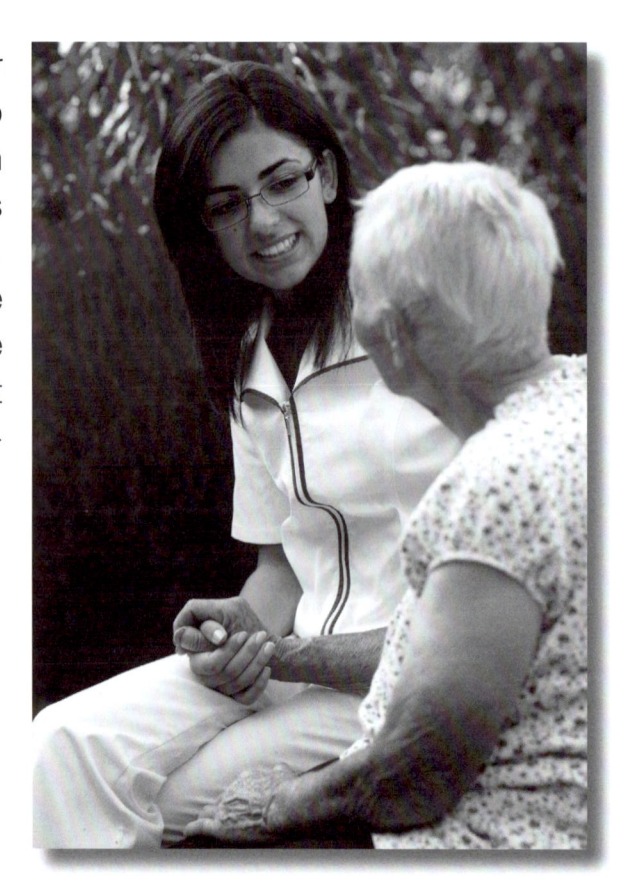

Hearing Loss

Permanent acquired hearing loss of a significant degree affects one in 12 of the adult population in Ireland. In the over-70 age group this rises to some 50%. Thus, about a quarter of a million adults in Ireland will have a permanent hearing impairment (most often due to ageing and/or noise exposure) that affects their quality of life, communication, social activity and participation to varying degrees (www.irishhealth.com). Imagine what it would feel like if you could not hear birds singing, music or other sounds. Loss of hearing can have a major psychological impact on individuals and affect their quality of life and their sense of safety (Rees 2004), and it can lead to social isolation and depression. Healthcare assistants require excellent communication skills when working with a person with hearing loss. Here are some steps that will help enhance communication with someone who has experienced hearing loss.

- Make sure that hearing aids (if used) are turned on and working. Batteries generally need to be changed every four weeks.
- Speak clearly and evenly; make sure that your mouth can be seen, to facilitate lip reading.
- Use non-verbal cues such as facial expressions and gestures to enhance communication.
- Be aware of facial expressions and body language.
- Reduce background noise, such as radio and TV.
- If discussing a sensitive matter, it is essential to maintain privacy.

- Get the person's attention before speaking, e.g. by using appropriate touch.
- Never approach a person with a hearing deficit from behind.
- Face the person at the same level.
- Use a normal pitch and tone when speaking.
- Learn to use sign language.
- Repeat questions as necessary.
- Be prepared to write things down, especially any instructions about procedures.
- Check that the person has understood what you have said.
- Make colleagues aware that the person is hard of hearing.

(Rees 2004)

Sight Loss

Caring for an individual with partial sight, sight loss or visual impairment is complex. Helping a person with sight loss also requires skilled communication, using both verbal and non-verbal cues in a sensitive manner. In fact, the role of the HCA when caring for clients/service users with sight loss should be one of support and empowerment to enable them to maintain their independence by overcoming environmental, social and organisational barriers. The goal is to adopt person-centred approaches to care, using effective communication methods and challenging disabling and negative attitudes and beliefs towards people with sensory loss (Veselinova 2013).

Examples of good communication techniques under these circumstances include the following.

- Identify yourself clearly on entering the client/service user's room or as you approach them.
- Speak in a neutral tone and pitch.
- Engage the client/service user's attention before you speak; use touch to get their attention.
- Stand or sit within their field of vision.
- Ensure spectacles are clean and within easy reach.
- Ensure that call bells or emergency bells are within easy reach.
- Adequate orientation to a new environment is essential.
- To avoid accidents, make sure that all areas are free of objects with the potential to cause injury.
- Introduce the client/service user to other clients/service users.
- Always introduce yourself on arrival and inform the client/service user when you are leaving.
- Speak directly to the person with vision loss; do not talk over them to relatives, e.g. 'What does he want to drink?'
- At mealtimes describe the place setting and food arrangement on the plate in terms of a clock face, e.g. 'Your potatoes are at three o'clock', to promote client/service user's choice.

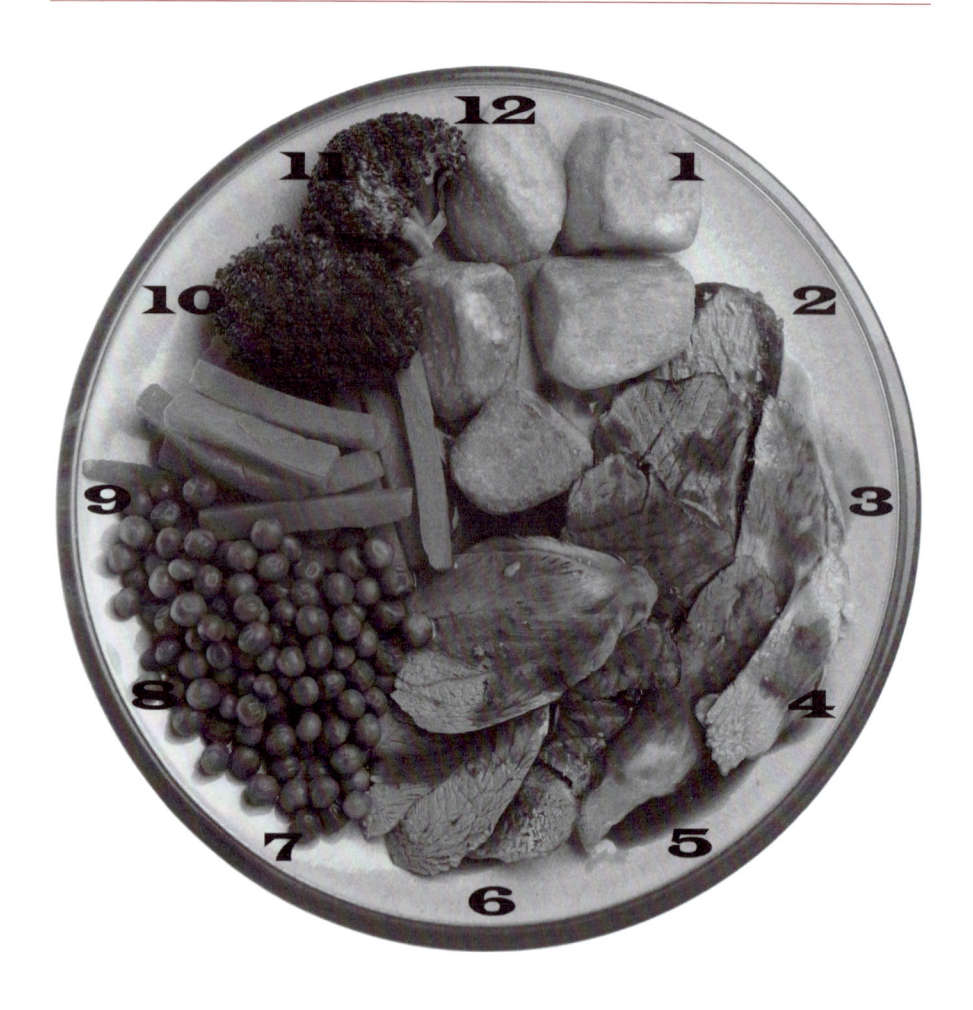

Loss of Speech

As a result of a stroke, for example, some clients/service users may have a form of aphasia and/or dysphasia, which is the loss of the ability to speak. Stroke is a major cause of speech loss; according to Nazarko (2004), every year 120,000 individuals worldwide experience a cerebral vascular accident or stroke. There are two types of aphasia: expressive aphasia and receptive aphasia. Incidentally, you may hear some similar terms being used in the care facility, but they have different meanings:

- *aphasia* – without speech (the prefix 'a' means without or unable)
- *dysphasia* – difficulty in speaking (the prefix 'dys' means difficulty with)
- *aphagia* – inability to swallow
- *dysphagia* – difficulty in swallowing.

Expressive aphasia: In expressive aphasia the intellect is not affected; therefore, it is very frustrating for the person, who knows what they want to say but cannot get the words out. Spending time with the client/service user and using communication aids, such as picture boards or pen and paper, may help. Remember not to speak to the person as though they are a child; reassurance and support is needed.

Receptive aphasia: There is impaired comprehension of the written and spoken word, even though the person can say the words out loud. They can see and hear words, but find it difficult to understand and remember, and they may use words out of context. Give assistance with re-learning the association between words and objects. Patience and time spent with the client/service user improves the outcome.

Communication difficulties following a stroke, particularly for those with expressive or receptive aphasia, can impede the patient's ability to communicate. Assessment and management advice from the speech and language therapist

(SALT) and occupational therapist can help promote means of effective communication and enhance outcomes for clients/service users (Matthews and Mitchell 2010).

Cognitive Impairment

Dementia is a term for a range of progressive, terminal organic brain diseases (National Audit Office 2007). The term 'dementia' is used to describe a collection of symptoms, including a decline in memory, reasoning and communication skills, and a gradual loss of skills needed to carry out daily activities. These symptoms are caused by structural and chemical changes in the brain as a result of physical diseases such as Alzheimer's disease (Nazarko 2009). People suffering from dementia commonly develop psychiatric symptoms first and later develop signs of cognitive impairment. Additionally, many individuals who have a cognitive impairment experience difficulties when attempting to communicate with and interact with others. People with dementia, whether as a result of Alzheimer's disease (AD), vascular dementia (VD) or Lewy body dementia (LBD), for example, often experience a deterioration of their communication abilities and it may be necessary for additional care and support to be provided in this area (Green 2012). When dealing with clients/service users suffering from cognitive impairment, particularly as a result of a dementia-related illness, there are a number of techniques the HCA can consider.

What Not To Do	What To Do
Argue with the client/service user – this will only cause further distress	Attempt to understand the client/service user's needs
Order the client/service user around	Remain positive
Compete with background noise, e.g. TV or radio	Speak slowly in a soft tone
Tell the client/service user what they cannot do	Avoid arguing, smile and make eye contact
Ask too many complex questions	Acknowledge the client/service user's opinions. Offer simple answers/choices and use closed questions
Treat the person like a child	Limit distractions
Approach from behind – a person with dementia is often easily startled/frightened	Allow for personal space

Remember, communication strategies that work for one person may not work for another. Similarly, the abilities of the person with dementia vary from day to day, so a flexible approach to communication is essential. As healthcare assistants get to know their clients/service users better, it is important to recognise the non-verbal cues indicating distress and over time to develop the ability to identify the factors causing this distress (e.g. fear, anxiety, pain, hunger or thirst). To communicate effectively and to deliver excellent person-centred care, the healthcare assistant must know their clients/service users as individuals. If you are employed or working in a residential care facility, refer to the individual's assessment 'A Key To Me' and/or try to discover the individual's 'life story' to get a sense of who they are and what their life story and meaningful activities entail.

THINK TANK

Knowing Yourself

How well do you know yourself? Stephen Covey (2004) defines self-awareness as the ability to think about one's thought processes and identifies that self-awareness is the reason why we can learn from our mistakes and, indeed, from the mistakes of others. Self-awareness permits us to examine how we see ourselves and to acknowledge how others see us. In fact, the majority of us are curious about how others view us and we often try to make sense of this through reflection.

While it is important to develop self-awareness, it is just as important to learn from experiences and consider the positive elements in every situation, no matter how difficult the experience has been (Duffy and Noone 2013). Take a few moments to think about yourself and answer the following questions.

- How do I describe my culture?
- How do I identify myself?

- Have I ever suffered discrimination? How did it make me feel?
- Have I ever judged someone only to find out that my initial perception was incorrect?
- In what ways can I non-verbally communicate my likes and dislikes to someone?

Now share your thoughts with the group and note the different and similar experiences and ideas on this area.

Visual Communication

TASK

A picture is worth a thousand words. Discuss.

Name some images and commercial symbols that come to mind when you think of this phrase. What is it that makes them memorable?

Images provoke thoughts and emotions in people; they stimulate discussion and convey meaning – all of this without writing a word. Galleries are full of thought-provoking images and artworks. This does not mean that images are better communication techniques than words; they are simply another method by which to communicate. Combining words and images often presents a very clear message – a tactic employed by newspapers with front-page news items. An understanding of the potential of images will help to enhance communication skills.

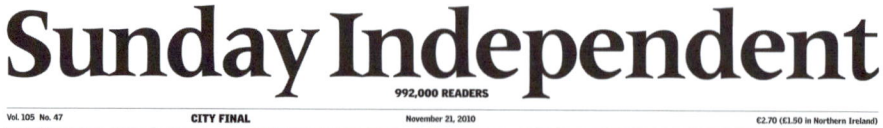

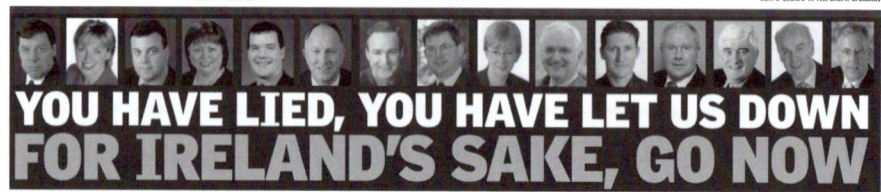

Visual Production

Being required to create a visual message can often cause worry as a person's lack of drawing skills or ability to use colour, for example, can make them feel limited. Nowadays, however, computer technology has made it much easier for us all to express ourselves using visual imagery. Couple the convenience of computers with the diversity of the internet and there is a vast bank of images to help people shape their ideas.

Posters and flyers: First choose a theme for the poster/flyer. Remember that text and imagery need to be balanced depending on the message you wish to communicate. Write down the objectives of the poster/flyer (limit to three aims). Perhaps write a small passage to accompany the poster,

Chapter 3 Non-Verbal and Visual Communication

describing it and the message in more detail. Think about who your target audience is. Choose an appropriate font style for the text.

TASK

Look at the anti-racism campaign posters below. Using a computer program such as Microsoft Word, construct an anti-prejudice campaign poster based on a prejudice that you have strong feelings about.

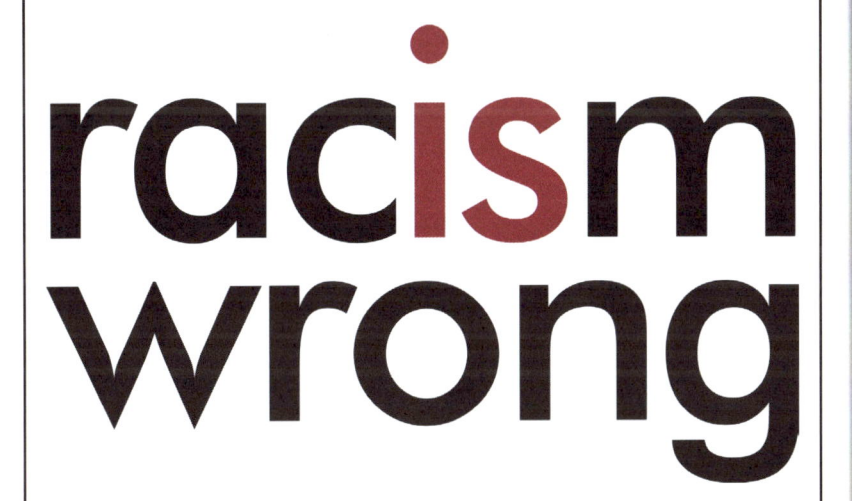

racism wrong

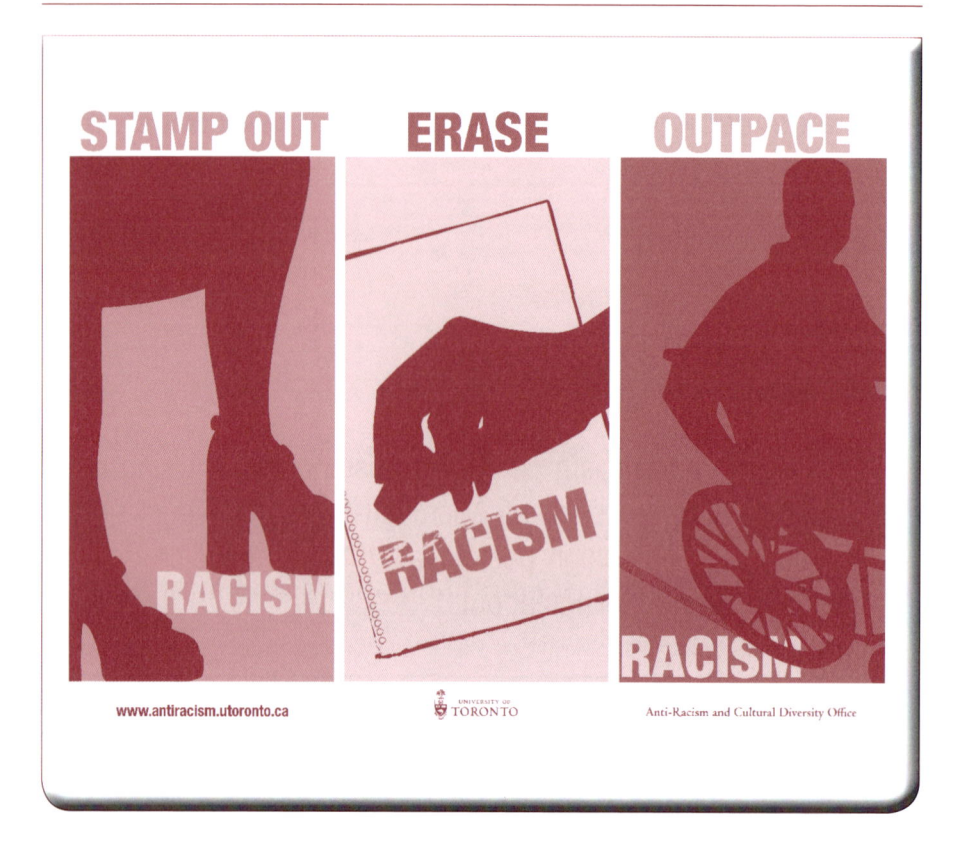

Communications for Healthcare

Chapter 4

Communications Technology

Chapter Outline

- Explain the impact of communications and information technology on personal, social and vocational life.

- Describe a range of communications technologies and their uses, such as the computer, telephone, facsimile, internet, electronic funds transfer, and data communications system.

- Use a range of communications technologies, such as email, fax and mobile phone, to exchange information with another person.

- Evaluate the advantages and disadvantages of the use of technology in communications.

- Outline current relevant legislation (the Data Protection Act and the Freedom of Information Act) in terms of rights, responsibilities, grievances and penalties.

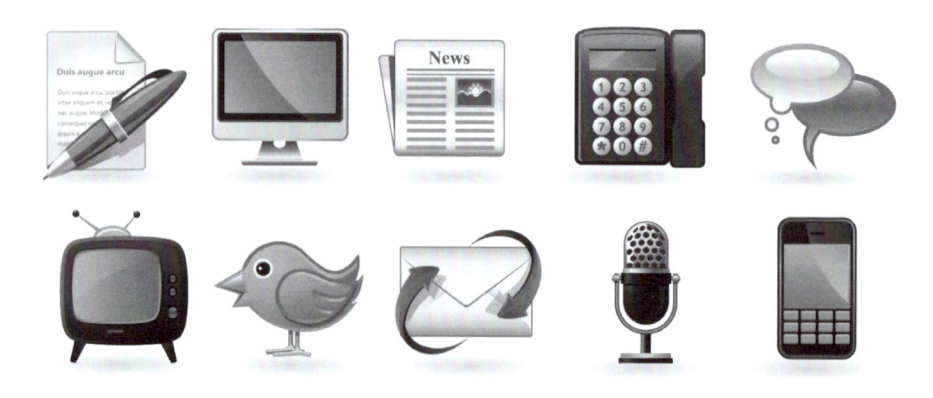

The Telephone

TASK

What are the differences between talking to someone on the telephone and talking to someone face to face?

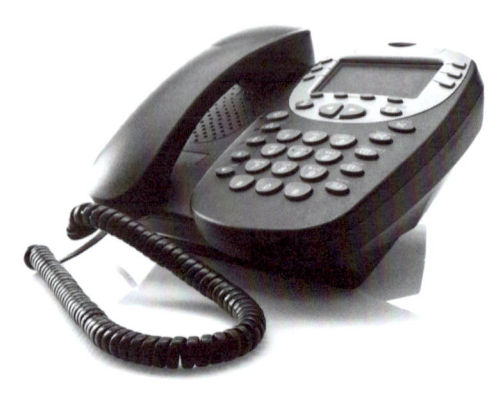

Technique: It is important to use the telephone effectively, especially in the workplace. Being aware of how to communicate a message to a receiver will enable you to understand good telephone technique. Improving telephone skills and manners is simple, and can help to avoid being misunderstood; it can also aid organisations to function smoothly as a team.

Here are some simple rules for using the telephone effectively.

1. Speak clearly.
2. Be clear about what you want to say and how you want to say it.
3. Have a pen and paper handy.
4. Make notes of the information you need to give or receive.
5. Be patient.
6. Be polite.
7. Use an appropriate tone of voice.
8. Be as efficient as possible – avoid delays.
9. Apologise for any delays you can't avoid.
10. Empathise with the caller.
11. Keep a record of calls.

Communications for Healthcare

TASK

There are pros and cons attached to each of the following ways of answering the phone – what are they? Discuss the suitability of each in social and vocational contexts.

- 'Hello' (use variations in tone)
- 'Hello, Drumlinn College of Further Education, Orla speaking'
- 'Drumlinn College of Further Education, Orla speaking, how can I help you?'
- 'Drumlinn College of Further Education, good morning'
- '11811'

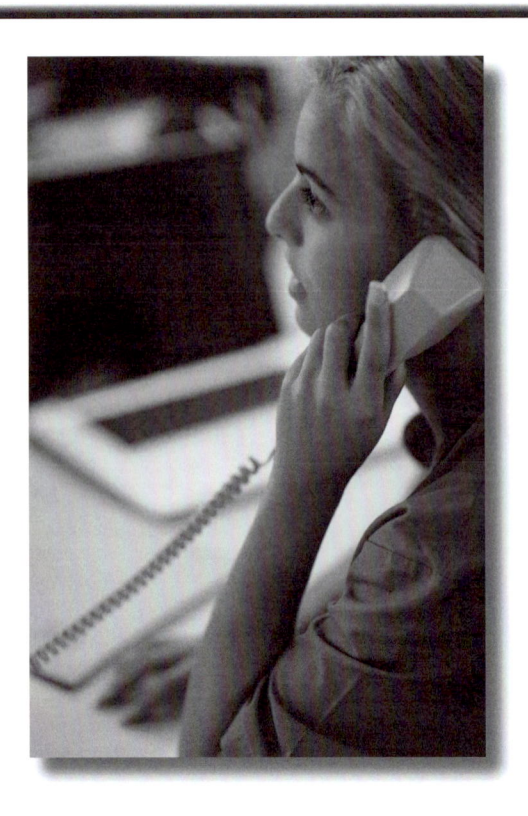

Leaving/taking messages: When taking a call, if the person asked for is unavailable, find out if anyone else can help; if not, take down the following information: who the message is for, the caller's name and organisation, caller's number, date and time of the call, reason for the call (i.e. the message), and your name.

It is common for messages to be recorded on sticky notes. Think about having a pen and paper available, and if messages are taken frequently, as at a reception, it may be a good idea to create a standard message slip such as the one below.

Message for: ....

Message: ....

....

....

Caller: ....

Of: ....

Number: ....

Time received: ....

Date: ....

Message taken by: ....

Communications for Healthcare

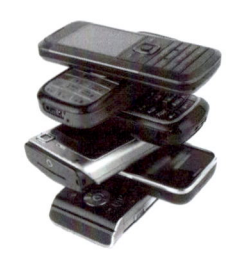

Mobile phones: The mobile phone is arguably the most successful new communication medium ever. Initially a mobile device used simply to have conversations, it has become much more versatile, encompassing access to the internet, texting, cameras and more – all on a small portable device. Furthermore, it is a piece of technology that rarely leaves a person's side.

TASK

Although the mobile phone has been a very successful creation, it can be intrusive in some social and work contexts. As a group, make a list of acceptable and unacceptable uses of the mobile phone, in both everyday life and the workplace.

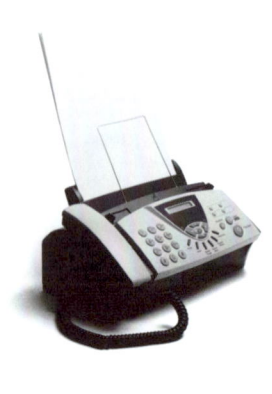

Fax: A fax machine is simply a long-distance photocopier which can send documents electronically via a telephone line to another machine anywhere in the world. It is gradually being replaced by email, but for the moment it is still in use. The sender dials the receiver's fax number and inserts the document into the machine, and a copy of the document is sent to the receiver for the price of a phone call. Sometimes a cover sheet is sent with the message; this usually includes details such as the sender's name, receiver's name, date, subject heading and whether it is a routine or urgent message.

Computers

People use computers in ways they may not even realise. In business, computers use bar codes and scanners to check customer credit, to check out goods at a supermarket and to check warehouse supplies. Electronic funds transfer (EFT) electronically moves funds (wages, bills) between bank accounts. Minute computers are embedded in many household electrical appliances, such as thermostats to control heating, security systems, clocks, radios, microwave cookers, DVD players and music players. Cars use computers to regulate the flow of fuel. Computers are used to control traffic lights and hospital equipment, book flights, fly aircraft and design anything from buildings to birthday cards.

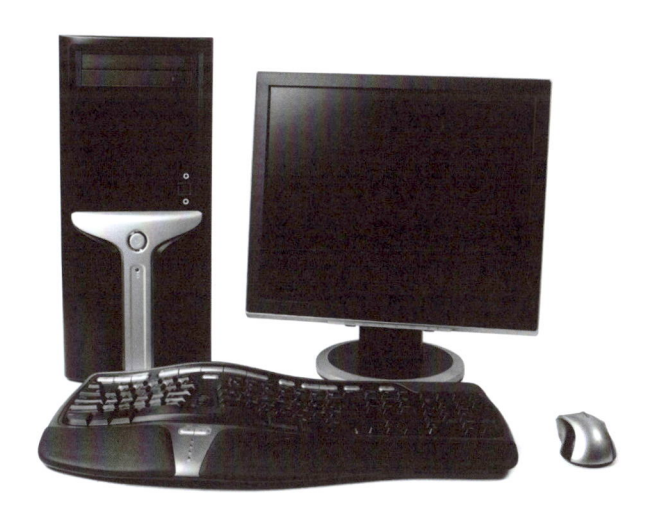

Most organisations use computers to keep files on accounts and personnel. At schools and colleges they are used to write reports and assignments, and design posters. Computers have become intrinsic to our lives.

An important aspect of law governs the way we deal with some types of information and data.

Freedom of Information

> The Freedom of Information Act 1997 as amended by the Freedom of Information (Amendment) Act 2003 obliges government departments, the Health Service Executive (HSE), local authorities and a range of other statutory agencies to publish information on their activities and to make citizens' personal information available to them.
>
> **Statutory rights:** In addition, the Freedom of Information Act establishes the following statutory rights: a legal right for each person to access information held by public bodies and government departments; a legal right for each person to have official information relating to himself/herself amended where it is incomplete, incorrect or misleading; and a legal right to obtain reasons for decisions affecting himself/herself.
>
> **Duties of public bodies:** Information about the activities of public bodies covered by the Freedom of Information Act (Sections 15 and 16) is contained in the Freedom of Information Manual which every public body is obliged to

publish. The information that must be made available in the manual includes:

1. A general outline of the structure and functions, powers and duties of the organisation; the services it provides to the public; and the procedures by which the public can avail of those services.
2. A description of the types of records held.
3. The arrangements made to enable people to access information and records, and to correct inaccurate or misleading personal information if this arises.
4. Information that may assist people to exercise their rights under the Freedom of Information Act.

In practice, most of the public bodies covered by the Freedom of Information Act have their Section 15 and 16 manuals available on their websites; paper copies of these documents are available, too. Also available is a list of public bodies covered by the Freedom of Information Act in Ireland. Since 31 May 2006 more than 100 additional bodies have become subject to the Freedom of Information legislation.

Requests for information: You can ask for the following records held by government departments or certain public bodies: any records relating to you personally (whenever they were created); and all other records created after 21 April 1998. A record can be a paper document, information held on computer, a printout, map, plan, microfilm, microfiche or audio-visual material.

Data Protection Commissioner: The Office of the Data Protection Commissioner is responsible for upholding the privacy rights of individuals in relation to the processing of their personal data. Data protection rights apply to information held on computer or in manual or paper files. These rights are contained in the Data Protection Acts 1988 and 2003. The Acts state that information about you must be accurate, only made available to those who should have it and only used for specified purposes. You have the right to access personal information relating to you and to have any errors corrected or, in some cases, have the information erased. If your information is being held for the purposes of direct marketing, you can have your details removed.

The Commissioner is an independent officer appointed by the government. Individuals who feel their rights are being infringed can complain to the Commissioner, who has powers to enforce the provisions of the Act. If the Data Protection Commissioner does not accept your complaint, you may appeal to the Circuit Court against the decision within 21 days. If you suffer damage as a result of a breach of your data protection rights, you may sue for damages through the courts.

The Commissioner also maintains a register, available for public inspection, giving general details about the data-handling practices of many important data controllers, such as government departments and state-sector bodies, financial institutions, and any person or organisation who keeps sensitive types of personal data.

See www.citizensinformation.ie.

The Internet

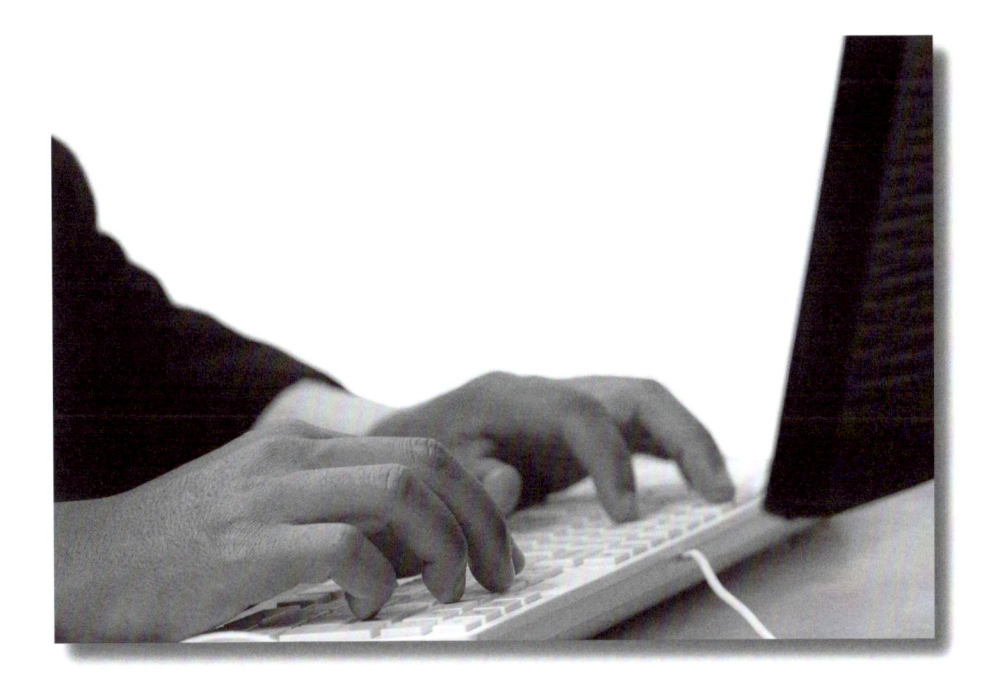

The internet is an **inter**national **net**work that links computers from all over the world and allows information to travel between them. Initially the concept was developed to allow easy sharing of academic information to aid research and development. With the development of the World Wide Web, it has become a global media-sharing phenomenon.

Communications for Healthcare

Survey

1. **Do you use the internet?**

    (a.) Yes

    b. No

2. **How often do you use the internet?**

    (a.) Several times a day

    b. Every day

    c. Several times a week

    d. Once a week

    e. Once a month or less

3. **Where do you use the internet? (Tick all that apply)**

    a. At home

    b. At work/college

    c. Internet café

    d. At a friend's house

    e. Library

    f. Other

4. **What do you use it for? (Tick all that apply)**

    a. Research/education

    b. Entertainment

    c. Shopping

d. Banking

   e. Travel/holidays

   f. News

   g. Sports

   h. Email

   i. Chat rooms

   f. Social networking

   g. Downloading music or videos

   h. Professional advice

   i. Other

5. **Are there certain types of website that you visit regularly?**

   a. Yes

   b. No

6. **What is the best thing about the internet?**

   a. Low cost

   b. Speed of communication

   c. Lack of censorship

   d. Worldwide access

   e. Variety of features/applications

   f. Other

7. **Which statement best describes your attitude to the internet?**

   a. A very useful source of information and means of communication

   b. A waste of time and only for nerds

   c. I'm addicted to the internet and use it even when I don't need to

   d. I have it at home but rarely use it

   e. I don't like the internet because I don't like technology

8. **Are you aware of the dangers of the internet?**

   a. Yes

   b. No

9. **Do you think that the internet should be censored/regulated?**

   a. Yes

   b. No

Using the Internet for Research

Here are some tips for using the internet as a research tool:

1. Write down the question or issue that you want to research.

2. Before searching, make a list of websites that might contain useful information and look at these first.

3. Scan each page quickly to see if it contains information relevant to your topic.

4. Copy the relevant information from each site into a single Microsoft Word document and save it.

5. Give yourself a set time for researching, perhaps 30 minutes or an hour. When the time is up, stop searching and revise your material, moving on to the next step of the process – mapping out the report.

> **TASK**
>
> Discuss the following topics in relation to the internet: data protection, freedom of information and copyright.

Email

In some ways a replication of normal postal mail, email is a communication technology that allows messages to be sent between computer accounts. It is cheaper and faster than conventional postal methods but without some of the usual formalities, such as home addresses and envelopes. First of all, though, you need a home – an email home, that is!

Email services are available from email clients such as Microsoft Outlook, Windows Live Mail, Gmail, Hotmail and Yahoo. The first two are used in a formal context and predominantly in business, whereas the last three are largely social mail servers. Signing up to these servers requires going online to the relevant server website and applying for an email address – a simple process which requires just a few minor personal details, such as name and address.

Sending/receiving: To write an email to someone, click on 'New Mail' or 'Compose' and a mail window will appear. There are two main sections: a header and a message. The header consists of a 'To' address bar to insert the recipient's address, a 'Cc' (carbon copy) address bar to insert any other recipients to be sent a copy of the message and a 'Bcc' (blind carbon copy) address bar, which means you can send the message to a number of people and those people only see their own address. There is a message title bar called 'Subject'.

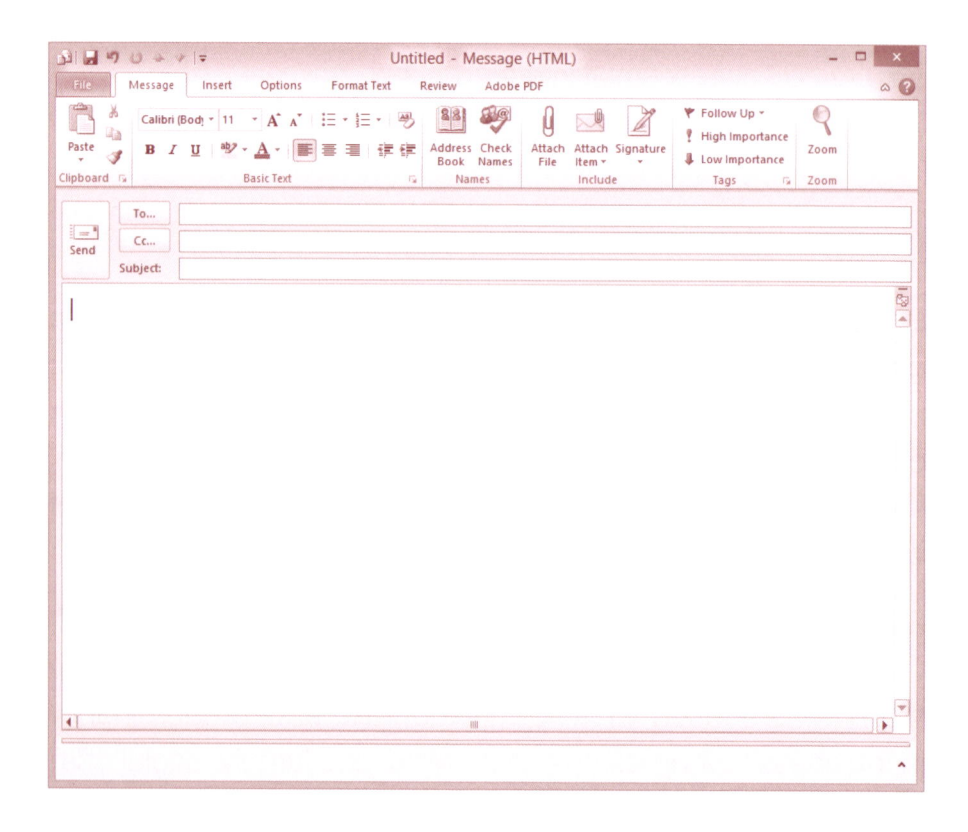

Underneath all this is the message window in which you type the body of your message. Signing off at the bottom of the mail follows the same rules for informal and formal letter writing.

To check for received mail, click on the 'Inbox' icon. A list of read and new unread mails will appear – double-click on any one of these to view the message in a new window.

Replying/forwarding/attachments: Replying to mails received can be completed very quickly. It is sensible to reply to a message immediately or as soon as possible after reading it. To pass on an email you have received to a different person, you can use the 'forward' option. This enables you to pass on messages to, for example, people who might be better able to deal with a query or who can bring the subject to the attention of another person.

Finally, it is possible to attach other files or images to accompany a mail message, such as a CV completed as a Microsoft Word document, or a holiday snap. A word of caution when receiving attachments: do not open attachments from senders you do not recognise. The email may contain a computer virus, which can affect the proper functioning of your computer.

Some final notes on emails: Be aware of company policies on the use of email in the workplace; be careful to make sure you send emails to the intended recipient; and pay attention to grammar in formal emails.

> **TASK**
>
> Send an email using all the functions described above.
>
> In groups, discuss the following issues: client knowledge, client rights, current knowledge, accuracy of information, electronic patient records, and monitoring clients and medications.

Appendix 1: Oral Presentation

Organising Your Presentation

Personal Considerations

- Wear comfortable clothes that make you feel good.
- Wear comfortable shoes that you are not likely to trip in.
- Decide whether you would prefer to stand or move around during your presentation.
- Prepare your voice.
- Prepare any cues to help the flow of the presentation.
- Make sure your material is well organised.
- Ensure your material clearly communicates your message.
- Follow the basic format of introduction, information giving, conclusion and question time.
- Address any concerns you have before the day of the presentation.

Practical Considerations

- The timing of each part of your presentation.
- Think of ways to help you stay focused, such as using pictures and notes.
- Is your topic well prepared?
- Do you require a drink to sip?
- Do you need help with settling nerves?

Presentation Outline

- Theme
- Introduction
- Areas of focus
- Signposting
- Evaluation
- Round-up of presentation
- Invitation for questions

Topic Selection

When considering a topic try to look at the following areas and choose something:

- you like
- with a lot of interesting points
- people will have an opinion about

- that is relevant
- that could transfer onto a picture/poster
- you know something about.

Visual Presentation

When designing a visual, ask yourself the following questions:

- Will I be able to represent my ideas in another way other than verbally?
- What colours reflect my topic?
- Should I use headlines?
- Will I focus mainly on pictures, mainly on words or a mixture of both?
- What do I want to include – data, concepts, jokes?
- Is this a do-able project or am I aiming too far out of my comfort zone? For example: if you are not an artist and dislike art, setting yourself a task of drawing will put unnecessary pressure on you.

How to Begin

The goal of pre-writing is to get what is already known onto paper. It is easily the most important step of the writing process. Once the bones of the paper (hopefully multiple pages) are laid out, start organising it and sorting out an outline of what the first draft will look like.

The first step of pre-writing is to put pen to paper, to realise what you know already and what you need to find out in order to write a concise paper. Once you are aware of the extent of your knowledge on the particular subject, you will need to do some research to fill any gaps that are left.

Researching a topic can take many forms, such as searching through a local library, conducting interviews or browsing a favourite search engine. The one golden rule of research is to make sure that the information gathered is both accurate and relevant to the topic. If the paper is meant to be mainly factual (not interpretive), try to use as many 'official' sources as possible. For example, information from the Central Statistics Office is far more valid than someone's rant on a personal blog.

Once a substantial amount of relevant research has been amassed, along with the writer's own experience on the topic, all that is left to do is to combine the two types of information. Balance is the key to this portion of pre-writing; too much or too little of either source of information may spell doom for the paper. So strike a comfortable equilibrium between personal ideas and the facts gathered from the research. One final note regarding research: always use references.

Many students have a problem starting the pre-writing stage. Sitting down with a blank document in front of you can be very intimidating, especially when there are no rules implied or stated, so do not feel bad if you are having trouble putting it together.

Outlining

One very effective way to begin free writing is by following an outline such as this:

Topic

Key idea #1
- Supporting idea A
- Supporting idea B

Key idea #2
- Supporting idea A
- Supporting idea B

Key idea #3
- Supporting idea A: detail 1, detail 2
- Supporting idea B: detail 1, detail 2

Note: Not all outlines will follow this format; this is merely a sample framework for beginning to organise your ideas.

Mind Maps

Another popular way to lay out ideas is by using a mind map, which is a simple diagram used to represent words, ideas, tasks and other items linked to and arranged radially around a central key word or idea. A common way to draw a mind map is with the main topic in the centre, and key ideas and their supporting ideas branching out from it. Think of it as an outline presented diagrammatically. The easiest way to begin is by getting a pencil and paper and drawing out your ideas, then connecting them.

Appendix 2: Assessment

Assessment Portfolio

The student is required to submit a collection of work that demonstrates evidence of the following communication skills.

Writing Skills

Evidence should include a range of relevant documents, including *a short structured report* and a *minimum of three other pieces*.

- The short structured report may be based on any topic, using information gathered from a variety of sources; it could be based on the candidate's vocational area or research done for another module (e.g. Work Experience Vocational Area Profile).

- A piece of personal writing such as short story/poem, letter of complaint/thanks/condolence/congratulations.

- Business documents such as a letter, memo, notice of meeting, agenda, minutes (narrative/action) or other relevant workplace documents.

The short structured report should be approximately 1000–1500 words and may be handwritten or word processed (refer to your college requirements). All the documents may be handwritten or word processed, but one item in your portfolio must be handwritten. Evidence of drafting, re-drafting and editing should be attached to at least one of the finished pieces.

Communications Technology Skills

Evidence of using information technology (IT) should be included, for example:

- Sending and receiving, both one-way (e.g. fax, answering machine and downloading information from the internet) and two-way (e.g. email and mobile phone).
- Display awareness of current and relevant issues, such as discussion of the uses, advantages/disadvantages and impact of communications technology; this may be a short written/oral piece and could be a topic for the report, oral presentation or discussion.

In one or more skills demonstrations, learners will be assessed in the following skills areas: listening and speaking skills, and visual communication skills.

Listening and Speaking Skills

Oral presentation skills: Candidates should make a presentation of approximately 5–10 minutes' duration. The presentation should be recorded on audio/video tape. The presentation may be on any topic of interest to the candidate. Ideally it should be on a vocational topic but may draw on other aspects of this module.

Dialogue skills: The ability to communicate one to one in a formal setting, such as on the telephone, in an interview, meeting, or question and answer session at the end of the oral presentation. The dialogue should be recorded on audio/video tape.

Discussion skills: These include non-verbal communication, listening and speaking skills. Candidates should participate in a formal group setting, such as a discussion or meeting. Evidence of the group interaction may be verified by the internal assessor.

Message taking/giving skills: Displaying knowledge of the communication process as well as information extracting, summarisation skills and message composing. Evidence should include original information in writing or on audio/video tape, or a message recorded on audio/video tape.

Visual Communication Skills

Candidates should communicate without words, either by:

- designing/producing (an) image(s) with or without text, such as a notice, poster, web page, brochure, flyer, greeting card, book cover, storyboard, video, flag, map, diagram, photograph, painting, sculpture, textile or sign; or

- communicating non-verbally and visually, such as making a non-verbal presentation using mime or dance, individually or in groups.

Evidence of development of ideas, with initial sketches, support studies and planning, to name a few, should be included. Evidence of visual communication may be incorporated into other skill demonstrations as visual aids or presented separately.

Grading

Pass: 50–64 per cent

Merit: 65–79 per cent

Distinction: 80–100 per cent

References

Ashmore, R. and Banks, D. (2002) 'Self-disclosure in adult and mental health students', *British Journal of Nursing* 11(3), 172–7

Bandura, A. (1977) 'Self-efficacy: toward a unifying theory of behavioral change', *Psychological Review* 84(2), 191–215

Burnard, P. and Gill, P. (2008) *Culture, Communication and Nursing* (Harlow: Pearson Education)

Burton, G. and Dimbleby, R. (2002) *More Than Words: An Introduction to Communication* (London: Routledge)

Covey, S.R. (2004) *The 7 Habits of Highly Effective People: Restoring the Character Ethic* (New York: Free Press)

Cowan, M., Maier, P. and Price, G. (2009) *Study Skills for Nursing and Healthcare Students* (Edinburgh: Pearson Education)

Duffy, A. and Noone, E. (2013) 'Writing a reflective assignment as a student HCA in Ireland', *British Journal of Healthcare Assistants* 7(7), 342–9

Goldsborough, D. (1970) 'On becoming non judgmental', *American Journal of Nursing* 2340–3

Green, D. (2012) 'Communication and cognitive impairment', *Nursing and Residential Care* 14(9), 446–9

Harvey, N. (2010) *Effective Communication* (Dublin: Gill & Macmillan)

Health Information and Quality Authority (HIQA) (2009) *National Quality Standards for Residential Care Settings for Older People in Ireland* (Cork/Dublin: HIQA)

Health and Safety Authority (HSA) (2014) *When and How Do I Report an Accident/Dangerous Occurrence*, http://www.hsa.ie/eng/Topics/Business_Licensing_and_Notification_Requirements/Accident_Incident_Reporting [accessed 1 September 2014]

Kalisch, B.J. (1971) 'An experiment in the development of empathy in nursing students', *Nursing Research* 20, 202–11

Kneale, J. and Santy, J. (2000) 'Orthopaedic nurses writing for publication', *Journal of Orthopaedic Nursing* 4(4), 185–90

Lewis, T. (2014) 'Communications and team working in peri-operative practice', *Journal of Operating Department Practitioners* 2(3), 139–44

Matthews, M. and Mitchell, E.A. (2010) 'Causes and rehabilitation of urinary incontinence after stroke: a literature review', *British Journal of Neuroscience Nursing* 6(1), 37–41

References

McCabe, C. and Timmins, F. (2006) *Communication Skills for Nursing Practice* (Basingstoke: Palgrave Macmillan)

National Audit Office (2007) *Improving Services and Support for People with Dementia*, http://www.nao.org.uk/wp-content/uploads/2007/07/0607604.pdf [accessed 4 September 2014]

Nazarko, L. (2004) 'Managing urinary incontinence after stroke', *Nursing and Residential Care* 6(12), 588–91

Nazarko, L. (2009) 'Advanced communication skills', *British Journal of Healthcare Assistants* 3(9), 449–52

Nicklin, P. and Kenworthy, N. (2000) *Teaching and Assessing in Nursing Practice: An Experiential Approach* (London: Ballière Tindall)

Nida, E.A. (1952) 'Selective listening', *Language Learning* 4(3–4), 92–101

Oxford Dictionaries (2014) online www.oxforddictionaries.com/definition/english/communicate [accessed 3 September 2014]

Rees, T. (2004) 'Hearing loss: causes, symptoms and communication', *Nursing and Residential Care* 6(1), 13–16

Stephenson, N. (2008) 'Self-directed learning: communication', *British Journal of Healthcare Assistants* 2(6), 301–3

Stonehouse, D. (2014) 'Communication and the support worker', *British Journal of Healthcare Assistants* 8(8): 394–7

Swann, J. (2009) 'Understanding vision part 1: structure and mechanics' *British Journal of Healthcare Assistants* 3(7), 318–22

Veselinova, C. (2013) 'Introductory awareness of sensory loss', *Nursing and Residential Care* 15(1), 8–12

Wood, J.T. (2007) *Interpersonal Communication: Everyday Encounters* (Boston, MA: Wadsworth)